Animals Before Breakfast

Also by Mary Bowring

The Animals Come First

Animals
Before Breakfast

Mary Bowring

W.H. ALLEN . LONDON
A Howard & Wyndham Company
1978

Printed and bound in Great Britain by
Billing & Sons Limited,
Guildford, London and Worcester
for the publisher, W.H. Allen & Co. Ltd.,
44 Hill Street, London W1X 8LB

ISBN 0 491 02425 8

Chapter One

My husband lay back in his armchair, stretched out his legs and gazed into the glowing log fire.

'This is the best way to celebrate New Year's Eve,' he said.

I nodded contentedly. Our son and daughter were at a party and we were on our own. We sat in the warm room in companionable silence having turned off the television. The only sounds were the slow ticking of the grandfather clock and the occasional crackle from the fire.

'I was thinking,' said Maurice reflectively, 'how, through all the years I've been a veterinary surgeon, all the times I've been called out at night and the social engagements that have been interrupted and often completely wrecked, somehow or other, we've always managed to see the New Year in together. Parties are all right, of course, but this is what I like most of all.' He glanced at the clock. 'An hour to go before midnight.'

We relapsed once more into a dreamy silence. Then, suddenly, the harsh ringing of the telephone made us both jump. We looked at each other in dismay then Maurice picked up the receiver, listened for a moment and said,

'I'll be right over.'

He looked at me ruefully. 'I spoke too soon, didn't I? It's a calving case. I'll never be back by midnight.'

I tried not to be downcast. 'Never mind,' I said, 'I'll wait up for you and we'll drink a toast when you get back.'

He stood for a moment looking down at the fire. Then, suddenly, 'Why not come with me?' he said. It's over at Harebell Farm.'

'What?' I stared at him. 'I'd love to come of course, but the Millers won't want me there at this time of night.'

'They'd understand. It's New Year's Eve remember.'

'It's a lovely idea,' I said, and rushed off to get my coat.

The country lanes were dark as we drove along but the stars glittered like diamonds over the frosty fields. Passing through the village we caught glimpses of brightly lit windows and warm rooms still hung with Christmas decorations.

I was glad we were going to Harebell Farm. If we couldn't celebrate at home there was no other couple I would rather spend midnight with than the Millers. Quiet, friendly people, they ran a small dairy farm and Maurice had been their vet for many years, so I knew we would get a warm welcome.

When we arrived the farmhouse was in darkness but the light was on in the calving box and I heard a murmur of voices as we approached. Then, as we entered I was delighted to see that Mrs Miller was there with her husband.

She greeted me with her usual broad smile. 'Now isn't this nice? We can keep each other company while the men get on with the work. Let's hope your husband can save the calf. Lily's been straining for nearly four hours.' She patted a bale of straw. 'Come and join me.'

I sat down beside her and gazed around with interest. It was like any other loose box, the floor deep in straw and a full hayrack in the corner but, at this time of night, it seemed strange and mysterious. A dim light, high up on a rafter and festooned with cobwebs, shone down onto a big black and white Friesian standing tied up to a ring in the wall. Deep shadows in the corners, the intermittent chirpings from several sparrows woken from their warm roosting place in the roof, and the two men standing looking at the cow, all seemed to create an atmosphere of hushed expectancy.

Then I heard Maurice ask Mr Miller, 'Have you felt inside?'

The other man shook his head. 'No. I thought it was all going to be straightforward. One of the feet came out about two hours ago but then it went back in again. Since then, although she keeps straining, nothing's happened and I can't get hold of anything to pull.'

'Just as well,' said Maurice, 'I expect the calf is lying all wrong.'

He took off his jacket, rolled up his sleeves and put on his long obstetric gown. Then, when he had washed his hands and arms in the bucket of water, he began to examine inside the cow. 'Yes. Here's the foot, but no sign of the other one. I expect—' he pushed his arm further in.— 'Ah! here it is. Folded back. I'll have to straighten it out. The head is lying right back, too.' He withdrew his arm and plunged it into the bucket. 'I'll have to give her an injection to stop the straining so that I can work the head forward.'

Mrs Miller looked at me. 'They'll be some time yet,' she said, 'Come into the house with me. If they haven't finished by midnight we'll take the drinks out to them.'

The kitchen was fragrant with the smell of warm mince pies and a large rich fruit cake stood in the middle of the table next to a bottle of whisky.

'I don't know what you think,' smiled Mrs Miller, 'but there's nothing I'd like better than a good hot cup of tea. We'll have it by the fire.'

She put on the kettle and I went into the living room, pausing for a moment in the doorway to admire the sight of the flickering firelight on the old oak beams. For hundreds of years these walls had sheltered farming families and echoed with the voices of generations of folk discussing the problems of their times. I sat down in one of the two armchairs standing invitingly close to the huge fireplace and let the warm peacefulness flow all over me.

Soon Mrs Miller came in with the tea and a plate of mince pies. 'You must have one. You now what they say every mince pie eaten before the New Year means a happy month.'

I laughed. Mrs Miller always had an old adage to suit the occasion. 'I've had so many already,' I said, 'I must be well insured by now.'

We sat there happily, exchanging local gossip until, suddenly she glanced at the clock. 'My goodness! It's ten to twelve. We'd better get out there right away.'

Armed with the whisky and glasses we went outside and, as we entered the calving box, we saw that the calf's birth was imminent. Two of the forelegs were already out and Maurice was easing out the head. He was dripping with perspiration and I knew that it must have been pretty hard going because, as a result of the local anaesthetic, the cow had not been able to help by straining, and he had had to haul the calf out inch by inch.

Without saying a word, Mrs Miller and I sat down on the straw bale and waited. Then, all at once, she held up her hand.

'Listen,' she said softly, 'the church bell is striking.'

We got up and stood at the open door looking out into the dark night and, from across the fields, we heard the solemn chimes.

'Eight, nine, ten,' counted Mrs Miller, 'eleven, tw—' and, at that very moment, there was a triumphant shout from behind us.

Turning quickly, we were just in time to see the calf fall onto the straw. For a few moments it lay perfectly still, then, as Maurice bent over it, we heard the first gasp of breath. Gently he dragged the little black and white bundle up to its mother's head, Mr Miller pulled the quick release knot on the rope and Lily looked down at her baby. Hesitantly, almost doubtfully, she gave it a little nudge and then, with a soft moo of pleasure, she began licking it all over with her rough tongue.

Maurice smiled with satisfaction. 'That will stimulate its breathing.' Then he turned to Mr Miller. 'A fine little heifer,' he said and stretched his back with a long sigh of relief.

The sight of the patient animal just beginning to feel the joy of motherhood brought a lump to my throat and then, as though to welcome this humble new life, the bells of the parish church burst into a joyous peal.

'A Happy New Year to us all,' said Mr Miller and reached out for the whisky.

Sipping the burning liquid slowly I turned to look at Maurice who raised his glass and smiled at me. A few minutes later as he put on his jacket he said, 'I'd like to wait until the calf gets up,' and Mr Miller nodded in agreement.

'Yes. We must make sure everything is all right.'

Gradually the little creature, stimulated by its mother's vigorous licking, began to rouse itself, and slowly turning its head, looked around for the first time at its strange new world. The soft, dark eyes gazed at us fearlessly. Then, at last, it began to struggle up. Soon it was standing on tottery legs and Lily gave a low moo of encouragement as it took a few uncertain steps to her side and began to search. Suddenly it found what it wanted and, this time, Lily's moo was deep with satisfaction.

We looked at each other and smiled.

'It's miraculous,' said Maurice, 'and it never ceases to amaze me. Without any guidance at all they know just where to look for their first drink.'

Mr Miller chuckled. 'Well, I know just where I'm going to have my second one. Come into the house and clean up properly. Then we'll have a little celebration.'

When at last we said goodbye, Mrs Miller laughed,

'They say that whatever you're doing at midnight on New Year's Eve, you'll be doing for the next twelve months so it looks as though you're in for a busy time.'

Maurice grinned at me as he opened the door of the car. 'Well, if all my cases end up like this,' he said, 'it's going to be a very enjoyable year.'

Chapter Two

The waiting room was full of people looking at their watches, but Maurice was not there to attend to their animals. He had been called out before breakfast to see a horse with colic and, although I had explained the situation to the clients, I was beginning to feel guilty at the sight of their reproachful faces. Obviously something had to be done to pacify them, so, drawing a deep breath, I decided to deal with some of the simple cases myself.

With the help of his master, I managed to clip the claws of an old dog, handed out some tablets to one or two clients and then, rashly, took on a long-haired cat belonging to a stout well-dressed lady who said he just needed 'a little comb-out'.

But when she placed the cat on the table, I looked at it in dismay. What should have been a beautiful half-Persian was a sorry sight indeed. Its fur, a dense mass of impenetrable tangles, looked like a grey, loosely knitted mat that had been put through a spin dryer.

'Can't comb her myself,' said the stout lady, 'she won't let me and I'd hate to hurt her. That's the worst of it when you love animals, isn't it? You can't bear to see them suffer, can you?'

'She's in a dreadful state,' I said at last. 'Cats are so particular about their fur. She must be very unhappy. Was she like this when you got her?'

Her owner sighed heavily. 'Oh! no. She was lovely and silky. But she wouldn't let me even brush her. She looks at me so angrily that I'm afraid she'll scratch me.'

I realised that I had taken on a hopeless task.

'I'm afraid I'll have to leave her until my husband gets

here,' I picked up the now furious puss and dropped her quickly into the basket 'I rather think she'll have to have an anaesthetic. Will you fetch her this evening?'

'An anaesthetic! Surely that's not necessary?'

'Mr Bowring will see what he can do, of course, but in any case it will take a long time.'

'It will cost me more,' she grumbled, 'still, I suppose it's got to be done. Well, bye-bye, Penny.' She waved her hand at the cat basket. 'Mother will come back soon.'

When I returned to the waiting room I saw, with a sinking heart, that every chair was taken. The latest arrival was a woman holding the lead of a small dog who sat, hunched and miserable, on the floor beside her. She caught my eye and pointed to her pet.

'My little dog can't do his wee-wee,' she said, and one or two of the other clients laughed. 'It's not funny—' She turned indignantly towards them, 'He's been like this for two days and he's in awful pain.' They stopped grinning and looked ashamed.

'He could burst his bladder and die,' said a man in the corner, glancing at me accusingly. 'He ought to be seen to at once.'

'Mr Bowring will be here as soon as he can,' I said and turned to the woman. 'You must come in first—' Then I heard the outer door open. 'I think he's here now.'

'Thank goodness!' I watched him putting on his overall and told him about the queue waiting outside. 'Is the horse better?' He nodded and I called in the client with the little dog.

'Poor old chap.' Maurice picked up his patient and put him on the table, 'Now, let's make you comfortable and get rid of that pain.' He signalled to me and we turned him upside down. I held him firmly and, luckily, he didn't struggle at all. Then Maurice gently pushed in a probe.

'There's the obstruction,' he said, 'Stones.'

Withdrawing the probe, he passed a catheter into the bladder and we watched as the urine poured into a bowl. When, at last, it stopped, Maurice said, 'There! I'll bet you feel a different dog.'

12

His mistress, watching anxiously, said, 'Will he be all right now?'

'No. I'm afraid not,' said Maurice. 'Those stones must be taken out. Has he had anything to eat this morning?'

She shook her head.

'Good. Well, I'll operate later this morning. You can fetch him this evening.' She went away comforted and the little dog settled down and went to sleep.

One after another the clients came in and we worked as fast as we could. As Maurice had begun his surgery so late it was lucky that most of the cases were straightforward. There were inoculations to be given, other injections, treatment for chills, dates fixed for future operations and small problems to be sorted out. Then, at last, I closed the waiting room door and Maurice opened the cat basket. Taking Penny firmly by the scruff he put her on the table and looked at her fur in disgust.

'What a mess! How could anyone let it get into such a state?'

'Her mistress said she loved her too much and was afraid of hurting her,' I said.

'Well, puss,' Maurice passed his hand over the cat's lumpy back, 'that's the kind of love you can do without. There's about a year's growth here. Impossible to get untangled without an anaesthetic.'

As soon as the cat was unconscious he set to work. Combing, pulling sticky lumps apart, cutting only where absolutely necessary, he gradually cleared his way through until there was a huge pile of matted fur on the table. It was a pleasure to see the comb pass smoothly all over the cat's body at last, just as she was beginning to come round from the anaesthetic. As we cleared up the mess, Maurice said, 'It always amazes me how many owners are literally afraid of their pets. Let's hope this cat won't be left uncombed again. Now we'd better get those stones out of the dog's bladder.' I put the instruments into the steriliser and got everything ready while Maurice examined his patient once more.

'Poor old boy,' I heard him say, 'I can sympathise with you, having had the same operation myself,' and I remembered the time, several years back, when Maurice had gone into hospital to undergo that very unpleasant experience. I remembered too the gruesome jokes he had shared with the doctors and nurses, comparing veterinary and human medicine, and the stoical way he endured the discomfort. As a convalescent, however, he left much to be desired, refusing to be cosseted and returning to work, in spite of my protests, almost immediately.

I came back from the past to find Maurice waiting for help. The anaesthetic given, we put our patient upside down again and the metal probe was put in and pushed up until it reached the stones. then, making a small incision of about half an inch, Maurice cut the muscle down onto the probe. With a pair of artery forceps he clamped back the sides of the urethra and then, using the 'crocodile' forceps, he began to pick out the stones. I looked at them with interest. There were four of them, very small, round and beige coloured, the largest being only about the size of a sweet-pea seed.

Taking off the clamps and giving an injection of antibiotic, Maurice said, 'The wound must be left open so that any further stones in the bladder can pass out with the urine. There are almost certainly some more higher up. It will only take two or three days to heal.' He looked at his watch. 'A good job I haven't many calls to make this morning. Perhaps now I'll have time to—' He was interrupted by the sound of the waiting room door opening and, when I went to look, I saw an elderly lady holding a small dog in her arms.

'Here—' She thrust the dog at me. 'He's scratching himself to death. I've tried everything but nothing works.' She glared up at Maurice who was standing in the doorway, 'And I don't suppose you'll be able to cure him either.' I was a little taken aback but Maurice smiled.

'I'm your last hope, am I? Well, let's see what I can do.'

The West Highland Terrier was certainly in a bad way. As I put him on the table I saw that there were inflamed patches all over his back and hindquarters. Even his tail was red and sore.

While Maurice was examining him I noticed that his client, a small rather odd-looking lady, with spiky grey hair

14

sticking out from under a hat like a pudding basin, was casting quick, apprehensive glances round the surgery and when, finally, her eyes met mine, she shook her head quickly in obvious disapproval. Then suddenly she said, 'I'm Mrs Lewis and I must tell you straight away that I don't believe in doctors for myself or vets for my dog. I'm a firm believer in Mother Nature.'

Completely nonplussed by this challenging statement, I glanced across at Maurice who looked up from his examination and said calmly,

'Well, Mother Nature hasn't helped much here. Your dog must have been scratching for months.'

'Yes, he has,' said Mrs Lewis, 'and no-one can say I've neglected him, because I've tried everything. Natural remedies of course. I don't hold with all these nasty drugs. I get advice from people who really know about animals – people like the milkman.'

'The milkman? I don't quite see the connection—'

'All those cows, of course,' she said impatiently. 'He was very helpful.' I saw Maurice's mouth twitch and I hastily turned a giggle into a cough when he said, 'That's interesting. What did he prescribe?'

'Well— milk, actually. He said it was the most soothing thing in the world. He told me to take five extra pints a day so that I could bathe Timothy in it and to let him drink as much as he wanted.'

'That must come a bit expensive. Has it made any difference?'

'Unfortunately not and, of course, my milk bill is enormous. Mind you, the milkman did warn me it might take a long time to clear the trouble up. I also asked my neighbour – her little boy keeps white mice – and she suggested dabbing on bicarbonate of soda but that didn't work. So then I asked a friend who used to live in South Africa and I felt sure she'd be able to help me. I mean, with all that wild life and lions and elephants everywhere—'. She paused, then added indignantly, 'To my surprise, she didn't know anything at all about animals. Just said I ought to take Timothy to a vet.'

'Best idea of the lot,' said Maurice drily, and lifting up the

15

dog's tail, he put a piece of cotton wool underneath and squeezed the anal glands, causing Timothy to give a little yelp.

'Oh! You've hurt him!' Mrs Lewis cried, 'Are you sure you know what you're doing?'

Maurice smiled. 'Don't get upset,' he said gently, 'It's all over. A simple little thing that has to be done when a dog's anal glands get blocked. They've been like this for some time and, of course, they irritated him intensely. He couldn't reach them so he scratched the nearest place and caused these sores. This eczema is self-inflicted.'

He picked up a syringe and gave the dog an injection. 'Now, that will stop the irritation very quickly and I'll give you some tablets of the same thing for you to continue the treatment for the next three or four days.'

'Pills! I don't believe in them—'

Maurice said patiently, 'You will when you see how quickly Timothy recovers. This is the way to get them down: take two pieces of meat and put the tablet in one piece. Give him that bit first while you show him the other. He'll gulp the first one down quickly in order to get the second. And those anal glands will need doing again in three or four month's time. You'll know when, because he'll begin nibbling at his back end. Bring him along straightaway and then you won't get this trouble again.'

Reluctantly Mrs Lewis opened her handbag. 'And how much will all that cost me?' she demanded.

'Not very much.' Maurice put the little dog on the floor. 'And don't forget to knock off those extra pints from the milkman. That should even things up a bit.'

He shut the door behind her and we gazed at each other in stunned silence for a few seconds.

'I think that calls for a strong coffee,' I said.

Maurice looked at me and grinned. 'Good idea. And how about some breakfast to go with it?' I stared at him. 'Of course! I'd completely forgotten you went out early to see that horse. You must be starving!'

'Your diagnosis is correct,' said Maurice.

16

Chapter Three

Living, as we do, in the South East of England, our winters are not on the whole severe. But we rarely escape entirely, and this particular morning the snow was falling steadily. As I stood gazing out over the garden I reflected that it was seen at its best from the window of a warm room and that, although it was undoubtedly beautiful, I still disliked it intensely. This was mainly because I worried about Maurice driving along dangerous roads and having to strip down in cowsheds or even out in the open. Not that he grumbled. It was just part of his life as a country vet, he said, and laughed when I fussed over him when he came home wet and cold. It was far better, he maintained, than working in a centrally heated office with 'flu and colds spreading from one person to another.

I turned away from watching the snowflakes and joined Maurice who was checking his case before going out on his weekly visit to our local Zoo.

He turned and looked at me. 'Are you coming?'

I hesitated. Usually eager to accompany him, I was slightly deterred by the weather but, before I could make up my mind, the telephone rang and I heard George, the Zoo Superintendent.

'Just thought I'd catch Mr Bowring before he sets out. Great news! A Polar bear has been born in the night. Unfortunately, Porgy – the male – was showing too much interest and Bess naturally was getting aggressive so we've had to take the baby away. We can't risk it being killed. We're going to try and rear it by hand.' I passed the receiver on to Maurice and he took down more details while I went to

17

put on my coat. No bad weather was going to stop me from seeing a newly born Polar bear and I was ready by the time Maurice had finished talking.

'I thought that would get you out,' he said. 'It's a great event at the Zoo and I only hope we can save the little creature. It's a shame it can't stay with its mother but, unfortunately, there's no separate accommodation for the male bear when a baby is born. This birth will undoubtedly decide them to build another den but it's too late for this particular one. George says everyone's desperately keen to see if it can be reared by hand though the chances are small.'

It had stopped snowing when we drove in through the Zoo gates and George came to meet us as we got out of the car. 'There's a casualty I'd like you to see first,' he said. 'It's a Rhesus monkey who has been in a fight and his family drove him right away from the warmth of the lamp. He's been in a very cold corner all night and he's pretty well paralysed, poor little chap.'

As we walked towards the monkeys' quarters I asked, 'Why do monkeys fight so much? They always seem to be attacking each other.'

'Well,' said George, always willing to enlighten my ignorance, 'in the natural state they live in colonies with separate family groups and, like all families, they fall out with each other from time to time. If one attacks another, the weaker one can run away and come back when the trouble's over. But in captivity there's nowhere for them to run so it's up to us to see they don't hurt each other badly.'

He led us into a small building and there, lying in a cage facing an electric fire, was a little greyish-brown monkey looking quite pathetic. Hunched up with his long arms clasped across his thin chest, his eyes were closed and he seemed to be in a coma.

Maurice opened the cage door, picked him up gently and examined him carefully. 'His temperature is still subnormal. It's going to take several hours to thaw him out properly. I'll give him an injection of heart and respiratory stimulant.'

George took the monkey in his arms while Maurice filled a syringe. Then, as he put the needle into the animal's thigh,

18

I saw the poor little creature half open his eyes. He closed them again as George put him back into the cage and Maurice said, 'That should perk him up a bit but I'll come back this afternoon and give him another one. He doesn't seem to have any bites on him but I expect he's been rather knocked about.'

George nodded. 'We can't leave him here too long or the others won't accept him back. Actually he's a very mischievous little chap. He has a habit of snatching people's spectacles if they come too close to the cage.' He grinned. 'We're always getting complaints from irate visitors but there's a warning up telling them not to go too near so if they lose their specs it's their own fault. Now come and see our important new arrival.'

He led us to the end of the block and there, in a very warm room, cuddled up in a box was a sight to make a child wild with longing. A miniature of its huge mother, it was only about eight inches long with white, slightly wavy fur, a little black pointed nose, a tiny head and rounded ears. Its eyes were not open of course, but when Maurice picked it up. It began to struggle and gave a high pitched demanding cry. Almost immediately a keeper came in holding a doll's feeding bottle containing a milky mixture, and stood waiting.

Maurice laughed. 'It's plain to see he's getting the VIP treatment. I'll just give him a vitamin injection then he can have his feed.' Soon the little bear was being cuddled like a baby in the keeper's arms and we watched as he sucked away vigorously with obvious pleasure.

'How did you get him away from his mother?' I asked.

'He was born in the den,' said George, 'but his mother came out to drive off her mate and she put him on the ground so we grabbed him through the bars. It was the only thing to do. Between the two of them it was in great danger. Whether it will survive now we just don't know.'

'The trouble is,' said Maurice, 'there really is no proper substitute for its mother's milk. That's where it would get the antibodies to fight infection. Also, of course, it has been born in abnormal conditions. In the natural state the mother bear is in hibernation when she gives birth, and when she wakes up her cub or cubs have already grown to a fair size and their eyes are open. Anyhow, I'll give it a vitamin injection every day for a while and we'll keep our fingers crossed. By the way, how is the mother taking her loss?'

'She's very uneasy,' said George. 'Keeps searching around and is very suspicious and hostile towards poor old Porgy. We'll certainly have to get the new enclosure built for him so that if and when she has another cub we can put him in there and she can rear her baby herself in peace.'

Soon the little one was fed and put back into his warm bed and, quite unable to resist my urge to touch it, I went over and stroked it gently. It was probably the only chance I would ever have to caress a Polar bear and, even though it was only eight inches long, it was still an unforgettable experience.

We went out into the snowy grounds. The Zoo was unusually quiet under its white mantle. Many of the animals were out of sight, sensibly lying in their heated dens and there were no visitors wandering around.

George said, 'Do you remember that terrible winter we had back in the sixties when we had masses of power cuts? We had great problems then.' He chuckled reminiscently. 'We worked out some wonderful schemes to keep the animals warm and fit and one of the funniest was giving the great apes a nightcap. We used to collect all the dregs from the glasses in the bar, add a bit extra to make up a sort of punch. Then, just before they went to bed, we gave the chimpanzees, orang-utans and gorillas a good long drink each. They simply loved it. Used to rub their tummies and grunt with delight. Then they reeled away into their dens to sleep it off. It was a good idea too. They survived the winter and kept cheerful into the bargain.' He turned to Maurice, 'By the way, I'd like you to look at the hippo. He's off his food and hasn't passed anything for twenty-four hours. We cleaned out his winter quarters a couple of days ago and put him outside while it was being done. There was a children's outing that day so I'm afraid it's the old story. Someone has probably thrown him some rubbish.'

The huge, ugly monster with his great broad head and tiny

protruding eyes was lying half submerged in his under-cover pool. 'I'll just nip back to the car and get my rubber boots,' said Maurice. A few minutes later he returned and opening his case he filled a jam jar with medicine. Then wading in towards the hippo, he said,

'Poor old Humphrey. Got a bit of indigestion, have you? Let's see what this will do.' He held the jar at the ready. 'Come on. Open up.' Bending down, he tickled the hippo under his chin and, to my amazement, Humphrey opened his great jaws. Quickly Maurice threw the liquid in and the enormous mouth closed up again.

'That's good,' said George, 'it means he's swallowed it. It's always a tricky job dosing a hippo. When he opens his mouth a valve closes to prevent him swallowing when he is under water and he could have ejected that medicine if he had wanted to.'

Suddenly I saw Humphrey give what seemed a great big yawn and then, to my horror, his jaws closed round Maurice's boot.

George saw my agitation. 'Don't worry. It's a favourite trick. Look—' I watched nervously as Maurice bent down and pushed gently at the hippo's mouth and, almost immediately, he was released. He walked out of the pool, grinning broadly.

'The first time he did that I was a bit worried,' he said, 'but he doesn't mean any harm. He just loves the taste of rubber, that's all.' He turned to George. 'Let me know how he goes on.'

Outside once more we went past the lions' compound and we stood for a few minutes watching as, invigorated by the wintry weather, these large animals played like kittens, stalking and pouncing on each other and rolling over and over in the snow. Then we moved away to watch the sea-lions playing with a big ball which they were tossing about in the water.

'They've had that ball for months,' said George. 'They rarely destroy any toy that floats and a piece of wood will keep them happy for hours. They throw it in the air, catch it

21

in their mouths, toss it into the water and dive after it. They really do play for the fun of it.'

'Don't all animals play, then?' I asked.

George shook his head. 'Some of them look as though they are but it's more likely that they're following their instincts for hunting and survival. Most of the 'games' played by the young carnivores are related to acquiring skill at finding and killing their prey. Other animals are learning to dodge to avoid their enemies.' He paused. 'Mind you, the more intelligent animals play. And in captivity they need quite sophisticated toys. Chimpanzees like rings, motor tyres and thing like that. Oil drums are great favourites and they work out simple ways of using them for their amusement. They bang them, make a terrific noise and then applaud each other by clapping their hands in glee. But, like babies, they're very destructive. And once they have developed a habit – good or bad – it's very difficult to distract them from it.'

'Of course,' said Maurice, 'animals in captivity don't have the constant struggle for existence so their energies have to find outlets in other ways.' He smiled. 'I remember some years back – before you came here, George – when Barbara the old elephant got bored and mischievous. She was on her own for a bit before the other elephant arrived and she was lonely. She pounded the eight-inch-thick concrete floor of her enclosure until it began to crack. Then she pulled pieces up with her trunk and, in a very short time, she had a hole about four feet across. While it was being repaired she had to be kept indoors so she reached up to the top of the wall with her trunk and started hauling out the bricks. She could easily have knocked the wall down by pushing up against it but she preferred to do it by taking out each brick individually. It occupied her mind. This went on for some time, alternately breaking up the concrete and pulling out the bricks, but when the young elephant arrived she was delighted to have company and immediately gave up the demolition game.'

George laughed. Then, pointing over towards the Polar bears' quarters, he asked, 'Would you like to have a look at Bess? Just to make sure she's all right?'

As we approached, it was plain to see that the mother bear

was still very uneasy. She was padding about from one end of the terrace to the other, sniffing into all the corners, returning to the den for a minute or two and emerging once more to continue her fruitless search. When her huge mate went near her she greeted him with angry growls and, not used to such behaviour, he took evasive action and plunged into the icy pool for a quiet swim while she went back to her vain quest.

'It's sad,' I said, full of pity for the poor bear and George nodded. 'Yes, it is,' he agreed, 'but if we had left the baby with her it would never have survived with the male around. As it is, she will have forgotten within twenty-four hours. She didn't have it long enough to get her maternal instinct really going.'

'She's perfectly fit anyway,' sid Maurice, 'for which I must admit I'm very thankful. Polar bears aren't exactly easy to treat. I well remember the first time I ever came into contact with them.' He chuckled and looked at me. 'You remember it, don't you?'

I certainly did. It was soon after he had bought this veterinary practice and, one day, a call came from the Zoo. Their official vet was retiring and they had a Dexter cow in trouble with a difficult calving. After Maurice had dealt with it satisfactorily, the Zoo manager had asked him to take on the job of looking after all their animals.

At first Maurice had demurred saying he knew plenty about cows but nothing at all about wild animals in captivity. Then, after a bit of persuasion, he agreed. In order to prepare himself he laid in a stock of books about wild life but, after studying a few, he put them aside having realised that there was only one way to learn and that was to study the animals themselves. By observing them when they were well he could then find out how to deal with them when they were sick. But when a message came that one of the Polar bears was off his food, he looked at me in consternation.

'The most dangerous and untrustworthy of all the animals there and it has to be my first patient,' he said. Then he grinned, 'Would you like to come with me and share my last hours?'

When we arrived we were told that these two fully grown

23

bears had only recently arrived from Moscow and had probably picked up some infection on the long rail and sea journey. They had been separated and the male, who was about eight feet long, was lying stretched out on the floor of his den looking very ill indeed.

Maurice looked at him for a long time then he turned to the keeper. 'That short, sharp breathing and the puffed out cheeks seem to me to be a typical case of advanced pneumonia,' he said. 'He must have been ill for several days. When did the trouble begin?'

'We don't really know,' was the reply, 'these wild animals tend to hide their sickness as long as possible. It's an instinctive fear of their own kind.'

'Well—' Maurice looked thoughtful, 'he must obviously have an antibiotic but he isn't eating and he drinks from that large pool so I'll have to give him an injection somehow. Can you arrange it so that I can have some control over him?' I nearly asked if he were going to give the bear an anaesthetic first but then I remembered that this would be fatal in a pneumonia case so I stood tense and nervous and resolved not to ask any questions at all.

The keepers were very resourceful and eventually decided on a scheme whereby they would get the bear into a passage leading from the den to the exterior. Then they would have to get a noose over a hind leg and pull him towards the bars.

When at last he was persuaded to go into the passage, a drop door was lowered at each end and they tried to get him to walk into a noose of rope on the end of a stick. But, having got to his feet, he was very suspicious and angry, growling ferociously and looking quite terrifying. I stood watching apprehensively, convinced that they would never succeed, when suddenly one of the keepers managed to distract the bear. He turned his head sharply, took a couple of steps forward and, in a flash, the loop of rope was round his leg. With their combined strength, the men managed to pull the huge creature down and towards the bars and Maurice reached through. Then my heart almost stopped as, just when he was about to give the injection, the bear jack-knifed over like lightning and his jaws clashed together just missing Maurice's arm.

'It was then,' said Maurice to George, having come to this part in his story, 'that I learnt however big and cumbersome a wild animal may appear, it will move with unbelievable speed when you least expect it. Anyhow, eventually we got the injection in and the bear improved, although each time he was due for another injection we had to think up new ways of distracting him. At the end of a week he was back on his food and appeared normal.'

'So he recovered then?' said George. But Maurice shook his head.

'No. A week later the pneumonia returned and he died within two days. I did a post mortem and found the real cause of the trouble. The poor animal had two fractured ribs, one of which had penetrated the right lung. Sometime during that long journey from Moscow there had been an accident. Perhaps the crate in which he travelled had been dropped or he might have been injured when he was being loaded up, we could only guess — but that was the cause of the pneumonia and the end had been inevitable. If I could have discovered the damaged ribs earlier he could have been painlessly destroyed, but of course a complete examination was impossible.' He looked at his watch. 'We must be off. I'll be back later today to give that monkey another injection and have a look at the baby bear.'

For a week the new arrival seemed to thrive and our hope rose. Each day when Maurice returned from the Zoo I demanded the latest news but on the seventh day he came home looking downcast.

'It was found dead this morning,' he said. 'Septicaemia caused by bacteria developing and lack of antibodies to resist infection. The artificial feeding was not an adequate substitute for the mother's milk.'

He poured himself a drink and then said thoughtfully, 'Remember that rather cranky woman in the surgery the other day with her theories about "natural remedies"? Well, in this case I'm bound to agree with her. Mother Nature knows best.'

I was having a peaceful afternoon. Maurice was out, vetting a horse, and the sun was shining so I decided to do some much needed gardening. I worked happily for half an hour when the sound of a car racing up the drive made me turn quickly. It pulled up in the yard and, as I went round to investigate, I saw a woman of about thirty-five get out leaving a schoolboy sitting in the passenger seat.

'A terrible accident—' she looked very distressed. 'Our dog has been run over. Is Mr Bowring here?'

'I think I can get him fairly quickly,' I said, 'Is the dog badly hurt?'

Her eyes filled with tears. 'I think he is dying but I haven't said so to Andrew.' She turned to look at the boy. 'He's got Barry on his lap.'

'Let me ring my husband immediately then,' I said. 'He's not far away.' Luckily there was someone at the stables and I waited impatiently while Maurice was being fetched.

I explained the emergency and he said, 'I'll be with you in ten minutes. Get the dog into the surgery – blankets, hot water bottle – you know the drill.'

I turned to the woman, who had followed me into the house.'I'm Mrs Redford,' she said. 'I was fetching Andrew from school when it happened—'

'Tell me about it later,' I interrupted, 'let's see to the dog first.' Going round to the side of the car I opened the door and looked at the boy, his face wet with tears, who sat with his arms round an unconscious Basset Hound. 'Will you let me take him?' I asked, but he shook his head. 'I can manage.'

Slowly and carefully he got out staggering a bit under the

weight. He was about ten or eleven years old, and obviously suffering from shock and fear for his beloved dog. Soon we had the pathetic bundle warmly wrapped up, and while the boy turned to his mother, I stole a quick look at the dog. He was not very old, about three-quarters grown, his gums were very pale and his breathing was rapid and shallow. There was a little blood round his mouth and his eyes were badly bruised but otherwise there was little to be seen.

Suddenly the boy broke down. 'It's all my fault! It's all my fault!' and his mother put her arms round him and rocked him gently to and fro.

'No, it isn't, Andrew. It wasn't anyone's fault. Barry has always had this habit of jumping out to greet you. You're not to blame.'

The boy lifted his head and stared at his dog. 'Do you think he'll die?'

There was an uneasy silence then his mother said, 'The vet will tell us. He'll be here in a few minutes.'

I put on the kettle, turned the gas up high and soon I was able to give them cups of strong tea into which I spooned a liberal helping of sugar.

'You must drink this,' I said.

Obediently Mrs Redford sipped the hot liquid but Andrew shook his head.

'You must,' I said firmly, and his mother added,

'Come along, darling, it will do you good.'

He sipped a little and then began to sob as if his heart would break. We looked at each other helplessly. At last I said, 'Try and finish the cup and then you can go and stroke Barry.'

While he was on his knees beside the still unconscious dog, Mrs Redford said, 'I was fetching Andrew from school but I couldn't park inside the gates as there was no room. I waited in the road and, as Andrew came towards the car, I opened the door to let him in. But Barry jumped over from the back and out onto the pavement. Then, in his excitement, he ran round the front of the car just as a lorry was passing.'

She stopped and Andrew began to say something but,

choked by tears, put his head down onto his dog and all I could hear was, 'Barry, oh Barry, please wake up.'

Mrs Redford recovered herself and looked at me pitifully. 'There wasn't a sound. Barry never cried out and I don't think the lorry driver even knew he'd hit anything. But the great front wheel hit Barry full in his side and he was lying quite still when we went to pick him up.' She lifted her head. 'Is that Mr Bowring's car?'

I nodded thankfully and, as Maurice pulled up, Andrew got to his feet and ran towards him.

'You'll save Barry, won't you? You won't let him die.'

Maurice put his arm round the boy for a moment. 'I'll do everything I can,' he said, and went over to examine the dog. I watched his face as he sounded the heart with his stethoscope, looked at the gums and watched the breathing. He took down a bottle of heart and respiratory stimulant and another one of blood coagulant and I knew then that there was internal bleeding. The two injections in, he stood looking down in silence and I saw Andrew gazing at him his eyes full of hope.

'He'll be all right, won't he?' And then, as Maurice did not answer, he said loudly, 'Aren't you going to do anything else?'

'Ssh! Andrew.' Mrs Redford held him tightly. 'Mr Bowring will do everything he can. He said so.'

Maurice turned and looked gravely at them. 'You're a brave boy, Andrew,' he said, 'and I'm going to tell you the truth. Now, your dog has been hit very badly and I think he's bleeding inwardly. That's what we call internal haemorrhage. It's very, very serious but he isn't suffering at all. I've given him an injection to keep his heart going and another one to try and stop the bleeding. Now I'm going to fix up a drip. This is to try and replace the blood which is leaking into his body.'

Andrew's sobs stopped as he watched Maurice take a bottle and, putting a length of rubber tubing onto the attachment, turn the bottle upside down to allow the liquid to flow. Then, pinching the end of the tube, he put a needle into the dog's vein and joined it to the tube. He stuck a piece of adhesive tape round it to stop the needle from coming out and hung the bottle on a hook in the wall just over the dog. We stood watching in silence looking at the bubbles coming up into the bottle and hoping and praying for some miracle to happen.

Maurice looked at Mrs Redford. 'There's nothing you can do here,' he said gently. 'Don't you think it would be better to take Andrew into the house with my wife?'

She nodded and moved towards the door but Andrew shook his head. 'I can't leave Barry – I must be here to see him come back to life.'

Maurice took his stethoscope again and listened to the dog's heart and, once more, looked at his gums and I could see that they were paler than ever, almost white, and his breathing was growing feebler.

He rose to his feet again and said, 'You mustn't hope too much, Andrew.' He drew Mrs Redford aside while I tried to engage the boy in talk but, listening with one ear, I heard Maurice say, 'I think the liver has been crushed. Do you think Andrew will be able to stand it when—?'

Mrs Redford's face went very white. 'I would rather he went into the house but he'll never trust you or anyone again if he isn't here all the time. He'll suspect you've put—' hastily she rephrased her words to confuse her son, 'used euthanasia.'

Maurice looked across at Andrew. 'You're probably right,' he said.

Andrew was answering me distractedly, his eyes never leaving the dog, and I longed to take him away from what I felt sure would soon come. I looked at his mother and then went to pour out some more tea which she drank in silence.

Maurice looked at his watch. 'Half an hour. I'll give him another two injections.' But he was fighting a losing battle. Gradually the dog's breathing slowed down and grew less frequent and then, after another quarter of an hour, there was a long pause, one more breath and that was all.

Mrs Redford saw it before Andrew had realised what had happened and, putting her arms round him she hid his face against her. She looked across at Maurice, saw him pass his hand over his eyes and finally unfasten the drip.

She kissed her son's head and said quietly, 'Darling, Barry has gone. He never suffered at all. Now you must be very brave.'

We got them eventually into the house and Andrew, sobbing wildly, took without thinking the tablet Maurice gave him and drank the water in great gulps. Then, throwing himself into an armchair, he turned his face into the upholstery. Mrs Redford, her face set and pale, sat clasping her hands together, gradually getting herself under control.

'To think,' she said at last, 'that I set out so happily to fetch Andrew and now we've to go back without Barry.'

Andrew turned quickly to stare at her. 'We're not going to leave him here. Oh! Mummy, we can't! We must take him back and— and— bury him in the garden.'

His mother's eyes filled with tears again and then Maurice said quietly. 'I had a dog once who died just like yours. He was run over. He was our very first dog after the War and he was out in the country with me and he put up a rabbit and chased after him. He ran through a hedge and on to a lane and at that moment a car came along and he was killed instantly. Like you, we were absolutely heartbroken. He was a young dog about the same age as Barry. We had no children then and he was everything to us. We buried him in our garden in his favourite spot between two apple trees and where we had a garden seat. And from that moment we turned that part of the garden into a very sad place. We used to go there and stand, always thinking of the lovely dog we had lost and feeling dreadful pangs of regret. After a while we got another dog – that's the only cure, you know – but we still could never sit under the apple trees without feeling unhappy. After three years we had to move away from that district and we simply hated leaving our dog there but it had to be done. Andrew—' he paused and the boy turned to look at him, 'take my advice and leave Barry here. Your mother, I'm sure, will get you another dog when you're ready for one. Oh! I know – you don't agree with me at the moment – but if you're a real dog lover you will never be quite happy without one.'

Mrs Redford said quietly, 'I suppose that's the answer.'

Suddenly Andrew glared at us all. 'How can you be so heartless talking about other dogs. There'll never be another one like Barry. I'll never forget him.'

'Of course you won't,' said Maurice. 'You wouldn't be much of a dog lover if you did. I've had lots of dogs and I've cried like you when they died. I can remember everything about each one. I'd love to have them all here with me right now. Where would dogs be if it weren't for people like us who give them good homes? Have you ever seen a stray dog? Poor, lonely creatures, longing for someone to give them affection. Dogs need us just as we need dogs.'

Mrs Redford got up. 'Now Andrew darling, we must go home. We'll leave Barry here for tonight, anyway, and think over what Mr Bowring has said.'

Maurice followed them to the door. 'I'll keep him until you let me know what you decide.'

We saw them off on their unhappy journey and, as the car went slowly down the drive, Maurice said, 'If only I could have saved that dog. But there it is – a very sad afternoon.'

Chapter Five

The circus loudspeaker blared out the time of the next performance and the laughter of children mingled with the raucous music from the merry-go-round. At the far side of the Big Top Maurice and I followed the circus owner into the section marked 'Private' and went towards a loose box where a chestnut gelding stood sweating and stamping restlessly.

'Poor old Lucky Boy' said Mr Johnson. 'He hates missing a performance. It's meat and drink to him.'

Maurice watched as the horse, in a spasm of pain, lashed out, kicking the door with a thud. 'Steady now, old chap,' he said quietly, 'We'll soon have you better.'

'It's Tuesday I'm worried about,' said Mr Johnson. 'I only hope he'll be fit for—' he broke off as the gelding gave a short squeal and began to lie down. 'Get up now, get up!' he said sharply, and Lucky Boy pulled himself back on his feet.

'A very bad attack of colic indeed,' said Maurice. 'He's as tight as a drum. We must get a head collar on to stop him going down.' He opened his case, 'I'll give him an injection to relax him.'

Ten minutes later he stood back. 'That'll take about twenty minutes to work.' He turned to the circus owner. 'What was that about Tuesday? Something special on?'

'Handicapped children,' said Mr Johnson. 'Every year we give them a show to themselves and they all love Lucky Boy. I told them his history once and it seems to have created a bond between them.'

'I suppose it would.' Maurice looked thoughtful. 'He has

to fight his handicap, too. He was a fine racehorse once, wasn't he?'

'One of the best. But he's gone in the wind now. Can't do anything very violent over a long period, coughs easily and gets these bad attacks of colic.' Mr Johnson shook his head, 'He's never what you might call really fit.'

Lucky Boy stamped restlessly and Maurice said, 'Yes. We're talking about you, old chap. He's very intelligent, isn't he?'

'No doubt about that,' said the circus owner. 'He can learn a new routine in a week and he loves the ring and the applause. Those handicapped children go mad about him and he seems to rise to the heights when they start cheering.'

'Of course, a family circus like yours is just the thing for him,' I said. 'You certainly look after him well.'

'I'll say we do,' the circus owner grinned at me, 'Jenny, my daughter, sees to that. She thinks the world of him and he'd go through his act with her if he were nearly half-dead. She'd be here now only she's just getting over a nasty bout of flu. She reckons she'll be fit by Tuesday but I doubt if Lucky Boy will.'

'Let's see,' said Maurice. 'This is only Saturday. I don't see why we shouldn't get him right by then.' He paused, 'There's only one thing worrying me. With this degree of pain it could be a twist. Could you get me a bucket of hot water, soap and a towel? I'm going to examine him.'

Afterwards, as he stood washing his hands, he said thoughtfully, 'I don't think it is a twist. More likely a spasmodic colic.' He glanced at his watch, 'We must be off now but I'll look in again on my way home. In the meantime, keep him walking. Don't let him lie down if you can possibly help it.'

It was nearly two hours before we returned. As we went into the loose box we found, to our surprise, a girl of about sixteen years old, standing talking quietly to the gelding.

'Hello,' said Maurice, 'what are you doing out here? I thought you had flu?'

'I'm better,' she said briefly and continued to stroke Lucky Boy.

34

Maurice looked at her searchingly. 'You're not fit yet,' he said firmly. 'Now you just go back into the warm and leave this fellow to me.'

Jenny gave him a tremulous smile. 'He'll be all right, won't he? Promise you'll get him well.'

'I promise,' said Maurice, 'and you must take care of yourself too or you won't be fit for Tuesday.'

She gave Lucky Boy a last hug and, when she had gone, I said, 'You've taken a chance, haven't you?'

He nodded. 'Yes. I've taken a chance and now I've got to keep my word. Ah!—' he turned as the girl's father appeared round the door of the loose box, 'Mr Johnson, I think someone should stay with Lucky Boy all night and ring me at the slightest hint of any change for the worse. Who is it to be?'

The circus owner passed his hand over his face in a tired gesture and sat down heavily on a bale of straw.

'That's a bit awkward,' he said slowly. 'I'm very short-staffed at the moment owing to this flu. Come to think of it, I'm not feeling too crisp myself but I think I'll have to do it just the same.'

Maurice picked up his case. 'Well, ring me if you need any help and tell me at once if there's another onset of pain.'

It was getting on for eleven o'clock in the evening when the telephone rang.

'Lucky Boy is going down,' said Mr Johnson.

'I'll be right over,' said Maurice.

An hour later he rang me. 'I'm going to stay here,' he said. 'The horse is in great pain. I gave him another injection but when I asked Mr Johnson to hold his head and cover his eye on the side I was going to inject he began fumbling with the head collar and said he couldn't see what he was doing. He looked awful. He's obviously got this flu and all his best men are laid up too. I'll ring again later to see if anything urgent has come in.'

It was early dawn before he returned and, although he looked tired, he was smiling. 'A good night's work,' he said. 'We coaxed and calmed and kept Lucky Boy constantly on the move and, at last, he won the battle.'

'We?' I asked.

'Jenny,' said Maurice. 'I'd been there about an hour on my own when she brought me some coffee. She said she felt much better and asked if she could help. At first I said no, but when I saw how Lucky Boy pricked his ears and, even in the midst of his misery, managed to give her a little whicker of welcome, I changed my mind. Obviously she meant a lot to him so I told her to go ahead and get him to relax by giving him all the cosseting she could. It helped enormously. She kept very calm and confident too so he didn't sense any distress or fear.' He smiled. 'I told her we would try to get along on Tuesday to see the performance.'

'That'll be fun,' I said. 'We haven't been to a circus since the children were small.'

'It should be good,' said Maurice. 'Jenny and her horse are both thoroughbreds.'

Chapter Six

I sat at the breakfast table waiting for Maurice, who had been called out early to see a sick cow. Through the open door I looked on to the yard where our hens were pecking around and basking in the early morning sun. From the side of the barn came our latest brood of baby chicks hatched only three days ago and led by their very self-important mother. I counted them carefully. Sometimes, when they are so young, casualties occur, but happily all eight little golden balls of fluff were there.

Our hens lead what I suppose is the perfect life for their kind as they have freedom to wander over the fields, plenty of natural food, a twice daily scattering of corn and a warm barn in which to roost at night. Periodically they gather in hopeful clusters round the kitchen door awaiting household scraps and this is very good for my morale because I never feel guilty about wasted food, knowing it will eventually be turned into glorious eggs with yolks the colour of apricots.

Admittedly we have to search for those eggs because, with their natural secretiveness allied to a sense of complete freedom, the hens tend to ignore our carefully placed laying boxes. But the thrill of finding still warm eggs half hidden in bales of hay or little clumps of straw, is a childish pleasure that never palls.

Unfortunately all free living creatures have their enemies, and a hungry fox is a killer. Two years ago we had a beautiful cockerel we named Louis, the Sun King, a magnificent bird, standing tall and proud in his brilliant plumage. He looked after his harem devotedly, shepherding them across the fields, finding them good things to eat and crowing loudly to attract the stragglers. Like all cockerels he was extremely self-sacrificing, always waiting until the hens were well supplied with food before eating anything himself and, even if given a scrap by hand, allowing a greedy hen to snatch it from his beak.

But a cockerel cannot stand up to a bloodthirsty fox and one day, hearing strange noises from the yard, I opened the kitchen door to see Louis, minus his gorgeous tail feathers, standing almost hypnotised by a fierce, mangy looking vixen who had chased him down from the field. As soon as she saw me, she fled and Louis stalked off to hide in the hedge and recover from the shock. But, later that year, he led his hens into the tall, ripening corn and never returned.

In the end the vixen was outwitted by my son John, who caught sight of her as she was just about to pounce on some baby chicks she had already made orphans by killing their mother. Armed with his gun, he crept stealthily towards her, despatched her with one shot and later received a substantial reward from his grateful father.

My musings were interrupted as Maurice's car swept up the drive and the chickens scattered in all directions. As I went out to greet him I saw him lift something in his arms and watched in amazement as he put a small brown hen on the ground.

'Another life saved,' he grinned. 'A battery hen who has gone broody and would have been bumped off if I hadn't said I'd take her. She's never been out of a cage in her life — let's see what she makes of the great big world.'

A hen's face is not noteworthy for its expression but that little bird looked thunderstruck. She stood absolutely still, staring at the vast expanse before her, the green fields, gently waving trees and grass all around. Then, as the other hens appeared, she cowered against Maurice's legs.

'She's frightened,' I said and, sure enough, as we moved away a few yards she pattered quickly behind us. 'She's bound to be,' said Maurice, 'and the others will chase her around a bit at first. Pecking order always has to be established but it won't be long before they accept her. The difficulty will be for her to accept them. I expect the shock of this sudden entry into a whole new world will put her off being broody but I'll settle her in the barn with some corn and water. First of all though, we'll let her stay out here for a while.'

We went into the kitchen and sat down to a late breakfast, leaving the door open; and the little hen remained staring at the fields. Then, suddenly, she turned, saw us in the kitchen and rushed towards us. I threw out some crumbs but the other birds came up in a rush and surrounded her. The older ones came to peck her and, terrified, she fled right into the kitchen and stood close against Maurice's chair.

When Margaret and John came down she was still there and had gained enough courage to pick up the crumbs Maurice put on the floor.

Margaret was enraptured. 'She's lovely. Poor little thing. I wonder if she would let me pick her up.' To her delight, the little hen, instead of squawking and struggling, stayed perfectly still as Margaret stroked her feathers and cradled her in her arms.

'I think we'll call her Lucy,' said Maurice. 'Don't ask me why – she just looks like a Lucy. It will be interesting to see how she copes with freedom. She knows nothing of a hen's natural life.'

The next morning, when we opened the barn door, the chickens, led by our new cockerel, rushed outside, clustered round the grain thrown down for them then dashed off to the field to pick up the early insects and worms.

A few minutes later, Lucy came hesitatingly from behind a hay bale, a little more confident now but still wary of venturing outside. 'She's obviously stopped being broody,' said Maurice. 'This traumatic experience must have shaken her hormones up a bit. She's got such a lot to learn and she's never had to fend for herself. I'll give her some corn to start her off.'

It wasn't long before she was accepted by the others and soon she was copying them, taking dust baths, scratching at the ground for insects and searching for tasty bits of clover in the grass. But when the cockerel led them out on foraging trips, she hung back and preferred to stay near the kitchen door. She learnt to fly up and roost at night and snuggled close to the others in the corner of the barn; but she was always first out in the morning to welcome us when we opened the door.

Eventually she went broody again and settled into a coop with eight eggs.

To our dismay, she was clumsy and broke six of them. Others were placed beneath her but she still managed to crush them until only two remained intact. Then one morning, three weeks later, we heard little cheeps and saw that she was the proud mother of two fluffy babies, one yellow and one black.

Her pride in her rather undistinguished achievement was enormous. Fiercely protective, all her latent maternal instinct came to the fore and the other hens drew back in alarm as she puffed up her feathers and clucked furiously if they dared to approach. Even Maurice and Margaret were not allowed near her chicks at first and we watched with interest as she taught them all the things she had never been taught herself. She showed them how to forage for food, scratching up the earth and standing back while they fed on the insects she uncovered for them. Then, settling down in a sunny, sheltered corner, she would gather her two chicks under her wings and sit looking out at the great, wide world in complete contentment.

Rescued from the concentration camp, Lucy had discovered real life at last.

Chapter Seven

Maurice stood back and surveyed the surgery. 'Yes. I agree with you. It certainly needs tidying up. Let's do it now. I've got some time to spare.'

'Oh good!' I got out the cleaning materials. 'I don't want Sheila to see it like this.'

'I might have known! I thought you said you weren't going to fuss about your cousin's visit.'

'I'm trying not to,' I said, 'but I haven't seen her for ten years. I'd like everything to be in order, then I can relax and entertain her.'

Maurice paused in the middle of throwing out empty bottles. 'I don't think she expects to be entertained. She said in her letter that she just wants to share an ordinary day with us.'

'That's what I'm nervous about. We never seem to have what people would call "ordinary" days. Not that I'm complaining,' I added hastily, 'I like it that way. It makes life interesting but it isn't conducive to gracious living.'

'Well, we've been lucky so far,' said Maurice. 'I've got a quiet morning for once so I'll be able to have coffee with you both. We'll probably have a nice leisurely time and she'll be most impressed by our life style.'

I laughed but I still felt doubtful. Experience has taught me that days that begin quietly seldom end in tranquillity. Hoping that this one might perhaps be the exception, I set to work. Soon the surgery was in good order and we were just about to return to the house when the waiting room door opened and a man came in.

'Sorry to come out of surgery hours,' he said, 'but I'd like

41

my cat to have its feline enteritis injection and, if you don't mind, I'll leave her here as I've got to catch a train. My wife will fetch her this evening.'

He handed a cat basket to Maurice and turned to go. 'Oh! by the way—' He paused at the door, 'she's a bit wild. I've only just adopted her. She's been living out in the woods.'

Maurice put the basket on the table and, as I prepared the injection, he opened the lid. Then, to my horror, there was a blood-curdling screech, a flash of black and white and the cat took a flying leap off the table and shot across the room into a far corner where she crouched, hissing and spitting like a small tiger.

I reached up to shut the flap of the window and the cat took off again, jumped up on to the sink and stood looking round wildly for an escape route. Maurice made to grab her but she dodged and knocked over the steriliser sending it crashing to the ground and spilling water, instruments and soaking cotton wool all over the floor. Frantic now, she turned tail, sent a pile of neatly sorted papers flying in all directions and raced along the shelves scattering everything in her path. We waited helpless until at last she jumped down, took refuge under a bench and stood, eyes gleaming, tail waving furiously, ready to take on all contenders.

Suddenly, with one quick movement, Maurice grabbed the long bushy tail and I thought for a moment he had got control but this was no normal cat. In a flash, she wrapped her front feet round her tail, climbed up on herself and with another frightful screech, bit Maurice through the palm of his hand. Involuntarily he let go and she retreated once more under the bench.

I began to search in the heaped-up chaos for some antibiotic powder but Maurice shook his head. 'I'll see to it later. I'll have to use the dog catcher.'

Going into the store room he returned with a long piece of piping with a noose on the end. 'Get the injection ready,' he said and, holding down the piping with one foot, he flung the noose round the cat's neck and pulled it tight. Struggling wildly the astonished animal was dragged out and dumped unceremoniously into the basket and, when I had put in the injection, he slipped off the noose and slammed down the lid.

'Phew!' I shook my head unbelievingly and Maurice began to laugh, 'What did that man say about his crazy animal? "A bit wild?" That must be the understatement of the year!'

I didn't know whether to laugh or cry. Our beautifully tidy surgery looked as though it had been raided by terrorists. But it was no use bewailing the situation, so, silently we set to work again. We were so engrossed that we never heard the door open and it was not until I turned from sweeping up a pile of broken glass that I saw my cousin smiling at us.

She gazed in astonishment round the room and then said brightly, 'I hope you're not having a spring clean in my honour.'

It was not easy to convince her that the surgery was not usually in a such a squalid mess but eventually we settled down for a much needed cup of coffee and Sheila entertained us with family gossip. At last she paused and looked at us searchingly.

'Tell me something. What is it really like, living in the country? Do you ever yearn for the bright lights? Don't you get bored at times?'

Maurice smiled and glanced at me and I shook my head.

'Well, no. You see—'

I was interrupted by the telephone and, as I was sitting next to it, I picked up the receiver. I listened for a moment then turned to Maurice.

'It's the Zoo. They want some more Aureomycin. Will you drop some in as soon as possible.'

'A zoo. That sounds interesting,' said Sheila.

'Would you like to see it?' Maurice asked and she looked at me questioningly.

I nodded and smiled and soon we were in the car. It was a cold day with drizzling rain and I wondered for a moment if we were doing the right thing. Trudging round the Zoo in bad weather seemed a strange way to entertain a guest. However, I took comfort in the thought that it would help to

43

pass the time and hoped George would be able to escort us round.

He was waiting for us when we arrived and after a few words of greeting he said, 'I'm glad you came right away. We've just discovered that we've a bit of tiger trouble. Remember Karen? The one we reared on the bottle. Well, she's going to another Zoo next week so we took her out of the compound yesterday and put her in a cage next door to some young cubs that are also going. They're much wilder than she is, of course, having been brought up by their mother. Unfortunately Karen didn't know this and when she put her paw through the bars in a friendly sort of way, they pounced on it. Now the whole leg is swollen right up. I expect you'll want to give her an injection of antibiotic. She's still fairly approachable although she's more than a year old but we'll have to be careful.'

Sheila glanced at me and I tried to appear unconcerned. 'That should be interesting,' I said calmly, and George laughed.

'I'm sure it will be. We haven't quite worked out how to deal with her so we'll have to play it off the cuff.'

The young tiger was lying down at the back of the cage and, as we drew near, she looked up and growled softly then began to lick her right foreleg as if to show us that she was in pain. The limb was badly swollen and almost twice its normal size and I saw Maurice frown as he looked at it closely. He turned to speak to the young keeper standing nearby.

'You're the one who reared her, aren't you? What do you suggest? Can I go in and inject her without getting torn to shreds?'

The man nodded cheerfully. 'I think so. She's still OK with me. I'll go in with you and make a fuss of her and, while I'm petting the sharp end, you should be able to get a jab into her hindquarters.'

I heard Sheila gasp and felt like doing the same, but determined not to let the side down, I hid my apprehension. Karen purred as the young man opened the cage door and went in followed by Maurice. She seemed relaxed and

44

friendly as her keeper stroked her head and spoke compassionately to her, and Maurice stood for a minute joining in the soothing talk.

'Why doesn't he get on with it?' Sheila whispered urgently, 'Surely it only takes a second to put in the needle?'

'It's not like that,' I said, 'He has to use a thick needle because of the tough skin so he must take it off the syringe, bang it in with a sharp blow – it's less painful that way – then fit on the syringe and push the plunger.'

'Oh my goodness!' She grabbed my arm as Maurice chose that moment to jab in the needle. But he got no further. Instantly Karen sprang to her full height – six feet at least – hit out at her keeper with her swollen paw and then whipped round and caught Maurice a blow with the other one. For one tense moment she hesitated. Then, snarling furiously, her golden eyes gleaming with anger, she laid down again and relaxed.

As the two men came out of the cage the keeper grinned at me and said, 'It's all right. That was just to tell us off for taking a liberty. Her claws were not extended.'

'I managed to get the needle out, thank goodness,' said Maurice. 'Now, how shall we go about it this time. She must have that injection.'

'Couldn't you dart her?' I asked hopefully, but he shook his head.

'Oh no! I wouldn't give an anaesthetic for a thing like that. Besides, it isn't necessary. She's not completely wild.' Wild enough, I thought, but said nothing and listened as the men discussed the situation.

At last the keeper said, 'I think if I go in holding something strange – a blanket perhaps – she will be so busy attacking it that you will be able to do your stuff. Let's try it, anyhow.'

The blanket was fetched and this time I found it difficult to hide my apprehension. Suppose — . But they were already in the cage, approaching the tigress very slowly and carefully.

As the keeper had predicted, Karen rose quickly to her feet, snarling distrustfully at this strange behaviour on the part of her friend, then she began to lash out furiously at the blanket which he held out to her. Immediately, Maurice lifted the corner and, bending down, stabbed the needle into her hindquarters. Engrossed in ripping and tearing the material she paid no attention and he quickly fitted on the syringe and pushed the plunger. A few seconds later I saw him nod to the keeper who dropped the blanket and followed Maurice out of the cage.

George chuckled. 'Nice work!' But we won't be able to fool her twice that way. We'll have to think up another scheme tomorrow.'

'I gave her a big dose,' said Maurice. 'Let's hope it will do the trick. Antibiotic in her drinking water may be enough.'

He looked at us then smiled at George. 'I think my wife and her cousin could do with a drink too. How about a quick one at the bar?'

'A very good idea,' said George. 'We'll—' he paused. 'What on earth is going on? Listen to that shouting – it's coming from the ape house.'

He turned to run up the slope and we followed on his heels. Suddenly he called over his shoulder,

'Good God! The gorilla has broken out!'

We stopped dead as we came in sight of a small crowd of agitated people huddled together and I could hardly believe my eyes. Umbi the male gorilla was standing in the open, staring at everybody in bewilderment. Then, as the crowd scattered, he turned and began walking on all fours towards us. It was a slow progress and we stood petrified as he lumbered along, his knuckles feeling the ground in front of him. Then, he suddenly changed direction and moved off sideways, down towards the bears' enclosure. A few more yards then he looked up, stopped, shook his head as if in disapproval at the rain and banged his long arms across his chest.

Maurice said, 'Poor old fellow. He evidently doesn't think much of this weather. Let's hope they get him back into the warm soon or he'll catch a chill.'

Two people with a small boy looking very shocked ran towards us and paused for breath. 'It's all right,' said

Maurice, 'Look – the keepers are surrounding him. What happened? Did you see him break out?'

The man nodded and pointed to the passage leading into the winter quarters of the large ape house where, in cold weather, the public can watch the inmates in their warm cages protected by strengthened glass picture windows.

'Jimmy was making faces at him,' he said, and the boy looked down guiltily. 'The gorilla threw himself against the glass and we thought it was rather funny. But suddenly he took a terrific run and crashed right through.'

His wife nodded, 'Terrible it was. There were several other people there and we ran for our lives.'

'He was frightened too,' said the boy. 'He wouldn't have hurt us.'

'That's all you know,' his mother said sharply. 'He might have torn us apart.'

Knowing Umbi to be a docile creature I thought this was most unlikely but Sheila said nervously, 'Don't you think we ought to get away. We don't want to meet him face to face.'

'Don't worry,' said Maurice. 'See – the keepers are crowding him. I expect they want him to head towards the isolation block.'

There were six or seven men around him now but, suddenly, he made a little rush at them and they backed quickly. Obviously worried, he turned his back and they approached once more and began to chivvy him gently along. Another man appeared from the other side of the ape house and Maurice said, 'I think that's Umbi's particular keeper. Perhaps he'll be able to persuade him to go in the right direction.'

'Oh! Look!' Sheila pointed. 'He's holding out his hand.'

We watched in amazement as Umbi, like a lost child relieved to find his mother, extended his long hairy arm, took the keeper's hand and walked quietly round the corner out of sight.

Five minutes later George came towards us looking very relieved. 'We've got him in at last. I don't think he's come to any harm but he's got a couple of cuts. One on the palm of his hand and one on a toe. You'd better have a look at them.

But first I'll show you how he got out.' He led us into the viewing passage and we stood aghast as we saw the great hole through which Umbi had crashed.

'That glass,' said George ruefully, 'is supposed to stand the weight of a full grown gorilla. We'll have to have an enquiry as to why it gave way.'

'What happened to his mate?' Maurice asked.

'Luckily she stayed in her corner. We've put her in with him in the temporary quarters. She's a bit fed up about it too. She likes watching him hurl himself around in the big cage. Still, as soon as the weather improves we'll get them both outside and that'll cheer them up.'

Going round to the isolation block we stood and looked at Umbi who was sitting near the bars, picking reflectively at a bunch of grapes. He seemed content to be back once more in warm surroundings and grunted with satisfaction as he gulped the grapes down but his mate sat sulking in a corner obviously disapproving as she looked the place up and down.

Maurice studied Umbi carefully. 'Nothing serious there,' he said. 'Antibiotic in his drinking water will do the trick and protect him against a possible chill. Now, how about a different kind of drink for us?'

It was while we were standing, glass in hand, being entertained by George with his repertoire of zoo stories that a call came over the loudspeaker for him to go to the office. He said goodbye and we went off on our own to look at the animals.

We were standing gazing at the sea-lions when he returned. 'We've just had a call for help and you are wanted as well. A Woolly monkey being kept as a pet has got out of its cage and, according to its owner, gone completely crazy. She has managed to trap it in the bathroom and wants us to take it away. It has bitten her dog so I told her you were here and she'd like you to attend to the poodle.

I was just about to suggest to Maurice that he should take us home first when Sheila looked at me delightedly and I realised that our unplanned entertainment was proving a great success.

George and a keeper led the way in a van and, as we drove

down the long drive leading to the Zoo gates, Sheila asked, 'What does a Woolly monkey look like?'

'Well, they come from South America,' said Maurice, 'and they're covered with a dense fur   rather like plush. They've got a thick muscular tail which they wrap round themselves when they're resting. Like most monkeys they can be vicious and, in my opinion, anyone who keeps one as a pet in an ordinary household wants his or her head examined.'

Soon we arrived at a small terrace house on the outskirts of our local town. The door was opened by a frightened-looking middle-aged woman who waved the men in quickly and then, as she waited for Maurice to get his case out of the car, she caught sight of Sheila and me.

'Won't you come in, too? I'm so nervous I could do with a little company. We'll shut ourselves in the kitchen so Willie won't be able to get at us.'

We followed her indoors and picking up a large teapot standing on the table she poured us a cup of tea each. Then she sighed heavily, 'Oh dear! I've had such a dreadful time. Willie belongs to my son and he's always looked after him because I'm too nervous to do things like cleaning out the cage. But he's gone abroad for some months and I thought I could manage although I wasn't too happy about it. How that monkey got out of his cage I'll never know but he scared me nearly to death, leaping all over the place. Then Peter my dog began barking and Willie flew at him and bit him and that was the last straw.'

The little poodle sitting in a basket in the corner looked cowed as Maurice examined him, searching carefully for a long time.

At last he said, 'No need to worry. The monkey hasn't drawn blood. It was more of a pinch than a bite. But I'll give him a dose of antibiotic just to be on the safe side.'

A few minutes later George entered the room looking extremely puzzled. 'I thought you said the monkey was in the bathroom, Mrs Wood. The room is empty.'

'Oh no! Surely not. He couldn't have got out   the window was closed.'

George scratched his head. 'Well, I don't understand it. We—'

Suddenly there was a shout from upstairs and he rushed back followed by Maurice who got through the door just before Mrs Wood slammed it shut. Listening anxiously we heard a muffled screeching and then we heard the men come downstairs. They went out to the van and a few seconds later George and Maurice returned and came into the kitchen.

George grinned rather sheepishly. 'He had us fooled. When we opened the bathroom the first time we could see nothing so we shut it again and looked in the other rooms. But the bathroom door opens inwards and Jim had the sense to look behind it and there was Willie hanging on the peg with one arm and looking like an old woolly jacket. We threw a sack over him and he's safely in the crate in the van. He's a bit cross so we'll be off right away.' He paused, 'You want us to keep him, don't you?'

'Oh! Yes, please.' Mrs Wood nodded vehemently, 'My son will understand. I'd never dare go near him again.'

Once more outside we peeped in the van and saw Willie huddled up in the crate, his thick tail wrapped round him protectively. He seemed to me to be a particularly ugly little creature, his face was round and fierce without the usual appealing look in his eyes that other monkeys have and he bared his teeth at us which made him even more unattractive. But Sheila was entranced.

'He's sweet. Poor little fellow. He'll be happier in the Zoo than in a tiny cage.' She reached forward to touch him but Maurice pulled her back quickly.

'Never, never do that,' he said. 'You could be badly bitten. Monkeys can carry all kinds of tropical diseases. I'm very wary of them. You can't be too careful.'

'My goodness!' said Sheila as she settled herself in our car. 'I've certainly had an exciting morning. Where to, now?'

'Home,' said Maurice firmly. 'I think it's time we had some lunch.'

I smiled to myself at Sheila's obvious enjoyment but I felt that Maurice would prefer to leave her with me for the afternoon. I was absorbed in planning a quick meal as we

50

turned into the drive leading to our house when I heard Maurice say,

'Oh dear! A client waiting for us.'

'A horse!' Sheila exclaimed. 'Standing right outside your kitchen door!' She beamed at me, 'Your life is full of variety.'

'It certainly is,' I said, and looked at the tall girl standing frowning impatiently as we pulled up.

'I've been waiting here for ages,' she said indignantly. 'My horse has been off his food for three days.'

'Three days!' Maurice stared at her. 'Why did you leave it so long?'

'Well, I thought he'd get better,' she said off-handedly.

I glanced at her in astonishment and even Sheila looked surprised. As we went into the kitchen she whispered to me, 'Do you think Maurice would mind if I watch while he examines the animal? That girl sounds awful – I'm quite intrigued.'

'I'm curious too,' I said, 'girls aren't usually so careless about their horses. In fact, they tend to go to the other extreme – worrying needlessly and rushing to the vet at the slightest little thing.'

The shaggy, ill-cared-for gelding stood quietly as Maurice took his temperature and, looking at the lack-lustre eyes, I was not surprised when I heard him say,

'It's a hundred and two point five. Did you ride him down here?'

The girl nodded indifferently and Maurice frowned. He took his stethoscope and after listening to the horse's lungs, he looked in his mouth, felt his throat for enlarged glands and studied the discharging nose. Then he said,

'I'll give him an injection then you must walk him back.'

'It's two miles!' said the girl indignantly.

'What of it? You should have consideration for your horse when he's ill. In any case,' – Maurice glanced at the girl's heavy figure – 'it will do you good. Now, put him in his stable and keep him there until I come tomorrow. Give him some bran mash if he wants it – something soft anyway – because his glands are up.'

Without so much as a 'thank you' the girl went off,

stumping angrily alongside her weary looking gelding and Sheila and I went back into the kitchen while Maurice remained outside watching. Suddenly he ran in and took his binoculars down from the shelf in the living room.

'What on earth—?' We followed him outside and as he put the glasses to his eyes, 'I'll bet she mounts that horse as soon as she thinks she's out of sight,' he said.

A minute later he exclaimed angrily,

'Yes. I knew it. I'll just go after her   shan't be long.'

He got quickly into his car and drove away and Sheila laughed, 'I wouldn't be in that girl's shoes for anything. Who is she?'

'I'm not sure,' I said, 'but I think she's the daughter of a man who has taken over a local farm and is making himself unpopular with everybody around. He's a rich businessman who has taken up farming for a hobby. We'll ask Maurice when he gets back.'

He returned rather red in the face. 'I read the riot act to her,' he said. 'She's walking the horse now. She was a bit rude at first but I think I got the message into her thick head. She's very like her father unfortunately.'

I nodded to Sheila and Maurice went on, 'He's a most unpleasant man. He is utterly ruthless when it comes to caring for animals but the girl may learn eventually. One of these days I shall tell her father to find himself another vet. I've only been there three times so far but each time we've had an argument.' He smiled at Sheila. 'One of the advantages of being self-employed – I needn't work for anyone I dislike. Within reason, of course, or we wouldn't survive for long.'

Sheila looked thoughtful. 'This morning has been an eye-opener for me. Is this a typical day for you?'

'Typical? Well, I don't know. Gorillas and monkeys don't escape every day but there's usually something interesting happening. Sometimes the animals are the problem, sometimes the owners. You meet a lot of people in this type of work, most of them nice, some of them foolish and a few – very few fortunately – positively objectionable. A fairly representative cross section of society I suppose.'

52

We had only just finished our lunch when, in answer to an urgent call from a farm, Maurice went off to see a cow and Sheila and I relaxed over our coffee. Not for long however for, as though to make up for our morning out, the telephone rang incessantly and I had to pass on messages for most of the afternoon.

At the end of the day, when we were sitting over a late meal, Sheila said suddenly, 'Well, I've made a big decision.' We stared at her in surprise and waited expectantly until she went on, 'I came down here to see if I could sort out a problem. David is going to have to retire early. His heart is none too good and he thinks it would be a good idea to get a cottage and live in the country. He's very keen but, up till today, I was convinced it would be deadly. But now that I've seen how you can live in the middle of the fields and still have an interesting life, I'm quite converted. But I've seen too that you must have something to do – something that will bring you into contact with people – so I've decided to start up a small business. I'm quite good at pottery – I've been to classes and I think I can branch out on my own. That way I'll still meet people – very necessary for me – and David can help without overtaxing his strength.'

From then on we discussed the pros and cons of her plan and when she got up to leave she looked pleased and happy at the prospect of a new life.

I felt pleased too as I waved goodbye. It was nice to know that we had been instrumental in helping her and I wished her well in her courageous new venture.

Back in the house we began to wash up and Maurice said, 'I don't know about you but I'll be glad to get to bed. It's been a pretty hectic day. I hope tomorrow will be quieter.' Then he began to chuckle. 'You know, it wasn't exactly an "ordinary" day, was it? A cat running amok, a stroppy tiger, a gorilla and a monkey on the loose to say nothing of horses, cows and the surgeries – Sheila will think it's like this all the time.'

I paused with a plate in my hand.

'Well – isn't it?' I asked.

Chapter Eight

I got up to pull the curtains and stood for a while at the window hoping to see the headlights of Maurice's car coming down the lane. He had been called out to see a horse and had been gone much longer than I expected. As always, my imagination was beginning to run away with me. I turned back into the room and rejoined John and Margaret who were sitting by the huge log fire watching television, quite oblivious, it seemed, to my nervous apprehension. Robert however, shared my feelings, looking up at me inquiringly as I stroked his silky head.

John said suddenly, his eyes still fixed on the screen, 'There's no need for you to keep jumping up and looking out of the window. Robert will know when Pop is coming, long before he turns into the lane.'

I nodded, wondering how it was that an animal could sense such things in advance. All our dogs had had the same uncanny accuracy in giving notice of their master's approach. However, there were no signs of happy anticipation at the moment so I tried to relax.

A moment or two later Margaret turned round. 'Robert's going mad,' she said.

Sure enough, he was standing by the door, whimpering and wagging his tail furiously. I let him out into the kitchen where he searched frantically for one of Maurice's slippers, and, holding it in his mouth, settled down by the outside door.

Returning to the window I waited. A few minutes later, I saw the flash of headlights across the fields and knew that once again, Robert's early warning system had worked.

Maurice came into the kitchen, bent down to take his slipper and shook his head at my offer of coffee.

'I think I'll have a whisky. It was icy out at Lockwood House.'

'Is the mare going to be all right?',

'Well, I hope so. I don't think it will turn to pneumonia.'

'How on earth did she get so chilled? She was in a stable, wasn't she?'

'That was half the trouble.' Maurice took his glass to the fire, 'She had been out in the field up to the onset of this extra cold weather and had grown a thick winter coat. Then they decided to bring her in and, foolishly, shut both the stable doors and put a thick blanket over her. So, of course, she got overheated, sweated too much – result – a severe chill.'

He sank into his armchair with a sigh of pleasure and Robert gave a final whimper of satisfaction and stretched himself luxuriantly at his master's feet.

'How is it that the dog knows long before we do that you are on your way home?' I asked. 'He was going silly, well before he could possibly have heard the car.'

'I suppose it's a kind of sixth sense. Dogs can read our minds a bit in things that concern them.'

Margaret laughed. 'I know that's true. I've tested it. The other day I had the biscuit tin on the table and I was helping myself from time to time. I also gave one or two to Robert. After a while he began to pester me for more and wouldn't leave me alone so I shut the lid. Then I looked at him and concentrated hard on a picture of the inside of the tin being completely empty. It worked. He stopped bothering and went and laid quietly in his bed.'

'Very scientific,' said Maurice, 'and next time, Margaret, when you are having a little snack and Robert is around, see if you can concentrate on a picture of me wearing a terrible frown at the thought of giving the dog fancy food. All the same,' he added, 'it is strange how, sometimes when I'm driving home with Robert beside me, I think to myself, "If there's nothing in I'll take the dog for a walk". As soon as we arrive, he waits patiently while you give me any messages or

I read something on the pad. Directly I decide whether I'm free or not he reacts accordingly, barks and gets excited or remains quiet. Of course, they can't read our minds in everything – it's only when they themselves are involved.'

The telephone broke into our conversation and I listened anxiously as Maurice answered.

'Good,' he said, 'and her breathing is easier? Fine. Well, I won't come over again tonight unless I hear from you.'

When he put down the receiver he said, 'They're very nice people. New clients. The house is lovely. Very old – I think it goes back to Tudor times. It reminds me of the place where I used to spend weekends before the War with the family of one of my school friends. It was haunted and in a most peculiar way too, because only the dogs saw the ghost.'

'Haunted?' Margaret and John pounced on the word, 'How? Who by?'

'Well, as the dogs couldn't talk we never found out. But it was really weird. I wouldn't have believed it if I hadn't seen what happened with my own eyes. We were having tea by the fire when I went to stay for the first time. There were several dogs there – two labradors, a terrier and my own Springer spaniel. They were lying on the floor in different parts of the room. It was a big room and they were quite far apart. Suddenly, in the middle of our conversation, they all rose slowly to their feet – my old Bill as well – growling, hackles rising, all staring in the same direction. Then, slowly, their eyes followed something that seemed to come from the far end of the room. They turned gradually, watched its progress over to the door, growled again, shook themselves and then laid down. My friends had watched my face, apparently, while this was going on and when I said, "For heaven's sake, what was that about?" they laughed. Then they told me that it went on every day at the same time. They'd got used to it but they were always interested when strange dogs arrived because they never failed to react in the same way. They said they had never felt any ghostly sensations themselves and that when the dogs weren't in the room no one was aware of anything unusual.'

Margaret shuddered. 'I'm glad there's nothing like that in this house. I should hate it if Robert saw ghosts.'

I bent forward to switch on the television but, once more, the telephone rang. It was only a request for advice and I sighed with relief as Maurice sat down again.

'I think,' I said thoughtfully, 'that in the far distant future, when we've all gone, this house will be haunted. By the telephone. Ghostly ringings and enquiries for the vet.'

'And a woman's face at the window waiting anxiously for him to come home,' grinned John.

'To say nothing of a ghostly dog running around with his master's slipper in his mouth,' said Margaret.

Maurice burst out laughing.

'What a picture of a veterinary family. Let's have the television on. There's a good animal film I'd like to see.' It will make a nice change.

Chapter Nine

'Last call of the morning,' said Maurice, as we drove out of our local town, 'and to a patient I don't much like. A fox.'

'Oh dear! Is it being kept as a pet?'

'Yes. These people – Foster is the name – found a cub in the woods. They decided it was an orphan and brought it home. Naturally their little girl fell in love with it. It's just over a year old now and beginning to smell to high heaven.'

'I suppose they look upon it as a kind of dog. You don't approve of that, do you?'

'I most certainly do not,' said Maurice emphatically. 'Foxes aren't dogs. They're wild creatures and shouldn't be confined in a domestic environment. This one can only be taken out on a lead and the rest of the time it lives indoors. It isn't even allowed to run free in the garden because it would escape – foxes can climb like cats and run up high walls.'

I was puzzled. 'But why do you object so strongly? You don't like foxes anyway.'

'Well – its funny. My feelings are very mixed. I dislike them for their natural characteristics – they love to kill, and not just for food. They get in a frenzy of blood lust and slaughter for the joy of it   but, of course, that's how they are and they can't help it. On the other hand, I hate to see an animal which is so wild and free being frustrated in all its natural instincts.'

He pulled up outside a house standing in a large garden.

'Would you like to see it? I'm going to give it an inoculation against distemper and hepatitis.'

A child of about ten years old stood on the doorstep and when she saw Maurice she called excitedly to her mother who was weeding the flower beds. Mrs Foster came forward smiling and led us into the house and, involuntarily, I wrinkled up my nose. The faint rank odour was unmistakable.

'Ferdy's in here.' She opened the door of a small room, showed us the dog basket in the corner and, at the sight of the little pointed face with its patches of white, the large ears erect and alert and the intelligent yellowy-golden eyes I forgot the smell and succumbed at once to the fox's charm.

'He's lovely,' I said and stroked the thick coat shading to deeper red down to its long brush; but he was wary of me and got up to prowl about the room.

Mrs Foster said quickly, 'Joanna, shut the door please,' and then, as I watched the fox roaming around and glancing up at the window, I felt a sharp pang of pity. Human love was no substitute for freedom where a wild animal like this was concerned.

The little girl took Ferdy by his smart leather collar, dragged him forward and, as soon as Maurice had given the injection, she lifted him into her arms and cuddled him protectively. Then, taking a ball from her pocket, she threw it across the room and the fox leapt down and raced after it.

As we stood watching them play together Maurice asked, 'Do you have any difficulties when you take him out for exercise?'

Mrs Foster laughed, 'Well, we get a lot of comments of course, but we don't take him far. He tries to slip his collar and we're frightened of dogs attacking him so we have to be very careful.'

'Hmm.' Maurice's thoughts were easy to read and Mrs Foster said, 'I know you don't approve, Mr Bowring, but what can we do? He seemed so helpless when we found him – we just couldn't leave him to die.'

Maurice said nothing. His eyes were following Ferdy who, tired of the ball game, was once more wandering restlessly round the room. It seemed to me that he was longing for fresh air, and the same thought must have occurred to Mrs Foster for she said, 'Joanna, put his lead on, darling, and take him for a little walk in the garden.'

60

Once they were outside, she turned to Maurice, 'You know, I'm getting worried about his smell. People tell me it will grow worse as Ferdy gets older. My husband thinks we'll have to fix up a kennel with a run in the garden. What do you think?'

'It's the best thing to do. The smell will certainly get worse – infinitely worse – and your friends will be reluctant to come into the house eventually.'

'I suppose,' she said slowly, 'we really ought to turn him loose in the country, though Joanna will be very upset if we do.'

Maurice shook his head. 'I don't think he'd survive long. You see, he has no fear of man now. He'd soon be shot or trapped and farm dogs would attack him if he went near them. I should build that run – take as much as you can spare from the garden – and give him as much exercise as possible. Anyway, I'm glad you decided to have him ino-culated. I'll give him his booster when its due.'

Back in the car I said, 'Poor Mrs Foster, she has a problem but you can't blame her for bringing the fox home. He must have looked so sweet and helpless as a cub.'

'He's equally helpless now,' said Maurice, 'and certainly not so sweet. But, as you say, one couldn't expect her to have him put painlessly to sleep. We shall just have to wait and see what happens.'

A fortnight later Maurice came home from his rounds. 'The Fosters have put Ferdy outside,' he said. 'He has a kennel, plenty of straw in it and a long run – the top is covered with wire mesh – so at least he's out in the fresh air. But he spends his time pacing up and down and just lives for his daily walk on the lead. Mrs Foster tells me they are going away for a week but their neighbour will look after the fox and will ring me if anything should go wrong.'

It was after several nights of heavy rain and cold winds that I answered the telephone and found myself talking to the Fosters' neighbour.

'Ferdy isn't well. He hasn't touched his food for two days and won't come out of his kennel. I've looked in and he's

61

shivering a lot. He must have stayed out in the rain and got chilled.'

I passed the message on to Maurice who was out on his rounds and, when he returned, I saw that he had a small cage in the car and soon, to my consternation, I saw Ferdy, wrapped warmly in a blanket and looking very sorry for himself.

'Had to bring him back with me,' Maurice explained rather sheepishly. 'That silly woman is quite incapable of looking after him and the poor little devil has got a very bad chill. I'll put him in the surgery. It's warm and dry and I can keep an eye on him.'

It was Maurice's half day so there was no evening surgery but next morning when I went in to help I stopped short in the doorway.

'Ugh! What a foul smell!'

Maurice looked up from his desk and grinned. 'I'm just writing this notice which I'm going to pin up in the waiting room to warn our clients and protect my reputation.' He held it out and I laughed as I read it.

'This unpleasant smell is due to the presence of a fox who is suffering from a bad chill. I hope it will be gone in a few days.'

'So do I,' I said fervently. 'I wish I still had my old wartime gas mask. How is Ferdy?'

'He'll recover. The antibiotic is working and he's taken a little raw egg and milk. I can't help wondering if I'm doing the right thing in saving him but I'm thinking of Joanna.'

Our first patient was a large Alsatian who began to growl as soon as he came into the room. Still on his lead, he tried to drag his owner to the cage where Ferdy lay but was headed off by Maurice and lifted protesting onto the table. A quick discussion of his symptoms, an injection and he was led unwillingly outside, to be followed by other patients who all reacted nervously to the alien presence in the corner. Our clients seemed highly amused though one or two held their handkerchiefs clutched to their noses and none of them showed any desire to stay longer than necessary.

I sighed with relief when the surgery hour was over. 'Poor Ferdy,' I said. 'He's not anyone's friend today.'

'He's mine,' said Maurice firmly, going over to his patient. 'He and I are building up a good relationship. Come on, old boy, take a little of this.' He held out a saucer of liquid and, from under the blanket, a pair of golden eyes looked out and a little black nose dipped into the mixture.

I looked at him closely and saw that his breathing was easier, then I said, 'Why, his eyes are just like a cat's eyes. When they meet the light the pupils contract into slits. Which family does he belong to? Dog or cat?'

'Neither.' Maurice gave Ferdy an affectionate pat and shut the cage door. 'A fox is a fox. They look rather like dogs, walk delicately like cats and have the same kind of eyes but they are unique.' He opened the windows, 'Like their smell.'

Ferdy made good progress and, by the time the Fosters returned, he was ready to go home. He still needed care and attention so they took him back indoors. Joanna was over-joyed but Mrs Foster was less enthusiastic and Mr Foster decided he had some urgent business that necessitated his staying up in town for a few days.

Then, a fortnight later, Mrs Foster telephoned. 'I don't know whether I'm glad or sorry but Ferdy has escaped. We put him back in his kennel a few days ago and next morning he had gone – burrowed under the wire. Joanna was terribly upset so I put some food out that evening and in the morning it was gone but nothing has been taken now for two days. Would you ask your husband to look out for him when he is on his rounds? Just in case he's got trapped or anything.'

We were both in the car, driving along a road with woods on either side when we found Ferdy. He lay cold and stiff in the gutter where he must have crawled after being hit by a passing car, and still wearing his smart collar. I felt a sharp pang at the sight of the pathetic, lonely little body and Maurice muttered something under his breath as he got out of the car and picked him up. Opening the car boot he laid him in and when he rejoined me he said, 'He was probably killed last night in the dark. He obviously had no intention of going back to the Fosters – it must be three miles at least from their house. I'll bury him in the woods when we get home.'

'I suppose you'd better tell Mrs Foster,' I said, 'then she can decide whether or not to tell Joanna.'

'I think the child should know the truth eventually,' said Maurice. 'It's the only way to help the young to understand Nature.'

'Supposing you had found Ferdy as a cub,' I asked curiously, 'what would you have done?'

Maurice thought for a moment then he said, 'I should probably have left him there in case his mother was around or put him painlessly to sleep. And you?'

Conjuring up a picture of an irresistible baby fox I said slowly, 'I'm afraid I should have done the same as the Fosters. Taken him home without thinking.'

'Hmm,' said Maurice and drove along in silence. When we arrived home he took Ferdy out of the back of the car and held him in his arms for a moment looking down at him.

'Poor little devil,' he said, and strode off to the woods.

Chapter Ten

'You'll never make it,' Margaret said incredulously. 'You know how bad you are at getting up in the morning.'

John agreed. 'She's even worse than I am. I'll bet you ten pence that Pop will go off alone.'

'I never bet on certainties,' said Margaret, then, turning to her father, she asked, 'Do you think Mummy really means what she says?'

'Of course she does,' Maurice grinned at our doubting offspring. 'If she wants to see me dart a stag and has to get up at 4.30 am to see me do it then she will.'

They went off shaking their heads and I laughed, 'They seem to think I'm a geriatric and incapable of making a little extra effort. But I wouldn't miss it for anything. I just hope it won't be raining.'

'I hope it won't be windy – it makes it more difficult to fire a dart accurately.'

'What is going to happen to the stag? Has it got to be treated for some illness?'

'Oh, no. Nothing like that,' Maurice explained. 'It has to be sent to another park where they want to introduce Red Deer. This stag will be followed the next day by three hinds to keep him company. In the autumn they will mate and this will gradually build up a new herd.'

'Why do you have to do the darting so early in the morning?'

'Well, the main reason is that the keepers have to get him over to the other side of London before the rush-hour traffic builds up. They don't want to be delayed on the journey because the stag might recover consciousness too soon, begin

65

to struggle and quite possibly damage his antlers. The deer are "in velvet" at the moment. Also the antidote must be got in as soon as possible because a highly nervous animal like a deer is very susceptible to shock.'

' "In velvet".' I pondered on the term. 'Do you know, although I've often heard it used, I'm ashamed to say I don't really know what it means.'

Maurice shook his head in mock disapproval of my ignorance. 'Deer shed their antlers completely in the very early spring. They start to regrow immediately but they look and feel quite different at first because they are enveloped in a sheath of – well – it can only be described as velvet. Gradually, round about July, this covering flakes off – you must have seen the long shreds hanging when the antlers have completed their growth and are bare and hard – and the deer are ready for the rutting season in autumn. When they are "in velvet" the antlers are soft and warm to the touch and very easily damaged so, tomorrow, before the stag is transported, they must be carefully protected by padding.'

It was a lovely May morning when we set out for the huge parkland where we were due to meet the gamekeeper. The sun had not yet risen and a silvery mist hung over the great avenue of chestnut trees as we drove in through the gates. Laden with white 'candles' they were in full bloom and, further on, enormous lime trees stood cool and fresh in their yellowy-green foliage. May bushes covered in sweet scented blossom looked like snowy hillocks and groups of deer turned their heads in mild curiosity as we passed. The keeper's cottage stood in a clearing with a small stream running along the front and a little bridge leading up to the gate and, when Maurice pulled up and we got out of the car, I stood for a moment drinking in the scene.

Everything was still, no breeze stirred the leaves and the air was sweet and scented. The bird chorus was greeting the day and in the background I could hear the soft cooing of wood pigeons, a sudden harsh call from a pheasant and, in the distance, the lovely echoing sound of the cuckoo – the theme song of Spring.

Maurice walked over to a stationary Land Rover and soon

66

we were greeting the Head Keeper, a tall grey-haired man, his son – a young man of about 21, and a dark, good-looking man of about forty who was the Under Keeper. They seemed rather surprised to see me but made me very welcome and I realised that Maurice had not told them I was coming. I gave him a quick glance but made no comment because the serious work of preparing the injection for the dart gun was about to begin.

We were all silent as we watched him measuring out the dose. The drug for anaesthetising animals is extremely dangerous and has to be handled with the greatest care. The antidote for man must always be ready for use in order to prevent a fatal accident. I was glad when, at last, the gun was ready and handed over to the Head Keeper who, by virtue of his position, was the one who had to select the stag and fire the dart. The weapon itself looked like a small shotgun and, climbing up into the Land Rover and sitting in the passenger seat in front, the Head Keeper held it across his knee. The Under Keeper took the wheel and Maurice and I, with the young man, went in the back. Then we set off, bumping across the grass in true safari style in search of a suitable stag.

In a few minutes we approached a group of about a dozen stags of various ages grazing quietly in the long grass and they looked up, suddenly wary, as our driver stopped and turned off the engine.

'That fellow there—' the Head Keeper said putting the dart gun slowly to his shoulder, 'just so long as he stands still.' Carefully he took aim then lowered it as the stag moved suddenly. 'Damn! He's off! He's suspicious.'

He turned to the Under Keeper. 'No use chasing him. He knows we're up to something. Let's find another.' We bumped on again towards another group and then, at about twenty-five yards' distance, the driver stopped.

'There's a fine one. A good red, too. He's about six years old.'

He was standing a little apart from a group of nine or ten of his fellows and he was undoubtedly the finest of them all. Quietly the Head Keeper took aim and suddenly – plop – I saw the dart hit the stag in the haunch. Startled, he galloped away for about fifty yards then he stopped dead and looked round to where the dart was clearly visible.

'Does it hurt him?' I asked, but Maurice shook his head.

'Not really. It's more like a dull blow. But he realises something has happened to him because he's beginning to feel strange already. See how the others sense it, too.'

We watched as the other stags followed, then closed up together and stood very still, like a crowd of curious spectators at a road accident.

'It will take a full ten minutes to work,' said Maurice and, as he spoke, the stag looked down at his side once more. The others drew nearer, ignoring us completely as we waited and talked quietly together in the Land Rover. It was almost eerie to see their steady concentration on the darted stag and the way in which he suddenly seemed to be an outcast. For a moment two of the young ones lost interest and began to spar with each other, standing up on their hind legs and looking rather like a pair of kangaroos. But, at a movement from the six year old, they turned quickly to focus once more their attention on their unfortunate elder.

'His hind legs are getting very wobbly,' said the Head Keeper, and Maurice nodded.

'Yes, but he's tough. I think he's fighting against the anaesthetic.'

'If the others were in full antler they would probably go and charge him now,' said the Under Keeper. 'But they know better than to do it when they're "in velvet". Ah! Look! he's going down.'

Slowly the stag collapsed as his hind legs gave way under him but, fighting hard, he reared himself up again. It was his last great effort however and gradually he sank down and lay stretched out on his side.

'Eleven minutes exactly,' said Maurice looking at his watch, 'but I think I'll have to give him a little more anaesthetic to make him last the journey.'

We got out of the Land Rover and went over towards the fallen stag and the Head Keeper said, 'I'll bet he's lying right on the dart.' As he went to retrieve it Maurice carefully filled a syringe and followed him. Luckily the dart was still visible and then, when Maurice put in the needle, I saw the stag close his eyes.

Suddenly the watching deer bounded away to a safe distance and, no longer interested, they began feeding again. As far as they were concerned it was all over with their companion and, probably, already forgotten.

As I joined the men the Head Keeper said, 'Feel his antlers, Mrs Bowring. You'll find it a strange sensation.'

I reached out and clasped one of the horse-shoe shaped points and was quite startled.

'Goodness! They're so soft and pliable. And they're almost hot.'

'That heat is caused by the copious blood supply that makes them grow so rapidly,' Maurice explained. 'The arteries will dry up as the antler hardens into horn.'

'Now, we must get on quickly,' said the Head Keeper. 'No time to waste. We've got a lot to do.'

The Land Rover drew up to the prostrate animal and a long wire cable was paid out from a winch which was fixed inside. Then the Head Keeper produced two wide leather straps and, drawing the front legs together, fastened the band. When he had done the same with the hind legs he covered each strap with sacking, securing that with a wire band complete with hook. That done, he hooked the cable onto the wire. The Under Keeper turned the handle of the winch and, with the son protecting the stag's head, he was carefully and slowly dragged up the ramp and laid on the floor of the Land Rover. He was well over six feet long and they had to bunch him up a little to get his head completely in. The Head Keeper's son grinned ruefully, 'Not much room for me. He's going to have a more comfortable journey than I am.'

Now great wads of cotton wool in gauze were brought out and the Head Keeper wrapped up each velvet antler from the tip right down to the round lump or 'boss' from which they grew and secured the protective covering with string.

'What would happen if his antlers were broken when he is "in velvet,"' I asked Maurice. 'Would he feel any discomfort?'

'Good gracious, yes. He'd be in great pain, they would bleed tremendously and, what's more, they would be deformed from then on.'

Standing there, watching the men working so quietly and skilfully, I reflected on how I had always taken deer for granted, admiring their graceful movements and their beauty but not finding them particularly interesting. Now, having touched the velvet antlers and learnt such a lot, I was filled with wonder at these strange animals.

The Head Keeper sat back on his knees and looked closely at the stag. 'There – I think he'll travel safely. Let's put this sacking under his face.'

His son pulled down the plastic cushions from the seats and placed them on either side of the animal and the father nodded approvingly, 'Good. He'll be well protected if we should have to make a sudden stop.'

'He looks very comfortable indeed,' I said, 'and listen – he's snoring away like mad!"

'Right! Now we must be off,' said the Head Keeper and, with the Under Keeper at the wheel and the son sitting inside with his hand on the stag's head, they waved goodbye, drove very slowly over the grass and headed towards the gates.

'Good luck!' we called, and stood watching for a while. Then we walked back to our car.

'What will happen at the end of their journey?' I asked.

'If all goes well it shouldn't take much more than three-quarters of an hour,' Maurice replied. 'And he will still be unconscious when they arrive. So they will unload him, the antidote will be given and he will be on his feet and feeding within two or three minutes.'

'And what about the hinds? Will you have to come at the same time tomorrow morning?'

'Oh no. There won't be any problems there. They have no antlers to protect. I shall go along after morning surgery, we'll select three, dart them, and put them into crates which will be fork-lifted onto a lorry. Then I shall inject the antidote immediately and they will be fully conscious for the journey.' He laughed. 'One of the few occasions when the female is not nearly as important as the male.'

70

As we got into the car I said, 'I'm awfully glad I came with you. It's been a most interesting experience and I wouldn't have missed it for worlds.' I looked at my watch. 'I expect John and Margaret will still be asleep when we get home.'

But we were greeted with the appetising smell of coffee and, looking rather pleased with themselves, they were preparing breakfast.

'How lovely to find it all ready,' I said gratefully and launched into a detailed description of our expedition. Then, as we sat down, 'It was well worth getting up so early. I wasn't so mad after all, was I?'

John grinned at his sister.

'Well, let's just say you're like Pop,' he said. 'Animal mad.'

Chapter Eleven

We were having an unpleasant week. Nothing was seriously wrong but little things were irritating us and we were both feeling rather depressed.

Shocked at the general state of chaos in the house, I had been obliged to do some late spring cleaning and found myself playing the house-proud tyrant, a role in which I am never very happy. Maurice had had his right thumb-nail crushed against an iron bar by an unruly cow and the nail was discoloured and loose, the small injury making things difficult for him when he was operating. Into the bargain, the weather seemed to have gone completely mad.

'Snow in May!' I exclaimed in disgust as I looked out of the surgery window and saw the blossoming trees covered in unwelcome snowflakes. 'We're back in winter again. How horrible!'

'It won't last long,' said Maurice, 'so stop grumbling and let's get on with this operation.'

The seven year old Border Collie bitch lying on the table had to have a mammary tumour removed and Maurice worked silently and quickly. But, when he began stitching up the wound, he muttered under his breath as his thumb nail caught in the fine nylon thread. I stood waiting, holding the roll of gauze ready for him to tie on and then, suddenly, I saw his face change.

'Quick!' he exclaimed. 'Heart stimulant – she's stopped breathing!'

I grabbed the bottle and syringe, measured out the amount and swiftly injected it into a muscle. Then, taking his stethoscope, Maurice placed it on the dog's chest and listened anxiously. After a few seconds, he shook his head and began giving artificial respiration and I watched in growing apprehension as he worked, pressing and releasing the ribs steadily and rhythmically.

Unable to bear the strain, I retreated into the office, leaving the door open so as to be within call, for it is at times like this that I realise my inadequacy. Even after years of work with Maurice I have never quite acquired the cool, calm efficiency necessary in emergencies and although I try to hide my nervousness, a mortifying feeling of panic is never far away.

I began to light a cigarette to steady myself, thought better of it, stubbed it out and sent up a kind of incoherent prayer. I was concentrating so hard on getting through to the other world that I started in alarm at the sound of Maurice's voice.

'The heart's beating again but very slowly.'

He looked up as I approached and something of my tension must have been apparent because he said, 'Stop worrying so! I think she's going to be all right. Another two cc's please.'

The injection in, he continued working for about a minute and a half until, at last, he exclaimed triumphantly,

'Firing on all cylinders!' and, heaving a long sigh of relief, he wiped his forehead.

'Thank God! That was a near thing.'

I gazed down at the Collie breathing steadily now, miraculously returned to life, and said gratefully, 'Yes. Thank God. I was praying hard.'

Maurice's eyebrows went up in astonishment. 'Is that what you were doing when you were in the office? Well! Well! Next time I won't bother to give artificial respiration I'll just get you on your knees. It will save me an enormous amount of trouble.'

He lifted the Collie, put her gently down on to a blanket, covered her with another and stood for a few moments watching her breathing. Then, turning to me, he held out his thumb nail.

'How about a spot of instantaneous healing?'

I burst out laughing and went to make the coffee but, at

74

that moment, there was a tap on the waiting-room door and Maurice went to investigate. When he returned he held the door open for a middle-aged lady who was being led in by a Labrador wearing the harness of a guide dog for the blind; and I recognised one of our favourite clients.

Mrs Perry, a widow living with her sister, had lost her sight many years ago. She never indulged in self-pity and we admired and respected her cheerfulness and courage. Not content with having adapted to her dark world, she went out of her way to help others who were similarly placed. She took long train journeys all over the country, giving lectures and visiting homes for the blind; and had made a full life for herself which, we knew, gave her great satisfaction.

As she bent down to take off the dog's harness, she said, 'I'm sorry I didn't manage to get here during surgery hours, but it is so wet and slippery underfoot that I had to go carefully.'

'You shouldn't have come out at all on a day like this,' said Maurice, 'I would have called with pleasure.'

'Oh! no. I like to have the walk and Bess needs the exercise. I'm going away tomorrow and I didn't want to miss her half-yearly check-up.'

Now that the harness was off I bent down to stroke the dog remembering a lesson I had learnt years ago. Out, one day, with John and Margaret when they were children, we had met another blind client and stopped to talk. The children, naturally, began to caress the dog but the owner, sensing this, said sharply, 'Never pet a guide dog when she is "on duty". At home I make a great fuss of her, but once her harness is on, she is working and mustn't be distracted.'

Maurice put Bess on the table and, while he did the routine examination, I gave Mrs Perry a cup of coffee. 'That's lovely,' she said gratefully. 'Now, I must tell you of something that happened the other day and made me rather worried. I took Bess for a walk in our local recreation ground when, suddenly, she stopped. I heard her crunching away and bent down to examine what she had found. Would you believe it – she was eating some small bones – chicken, I think. I felt around and found a piece of paper with what seemed to be a whole carcass of the bird. There are houses all along the edge of the recreation ground so I suppose some thoughtless person had just thrown the household rubbish over the fence. If only people realised the danger to dogs and, in particular, guide dogs, whose owners can't see what is lying around. Bess has been trained not to pick up anything at all but the temptation is very strong when things like that lie right in her path. It's made me wary of taking her there again. Chicken bones are dangerous, aren't they?'

'They certainly are,' said Maurice. 'Oh! I know you meet people who say their dog has never come to any harm in spite of being given splintery ones like lamb's ribs and poultry carcasses and, of course, some dogs are lucky enough to get away with it. But the risk is very real and should never be taken.'

He went on with his examination, checking everything to make sure Bess was perfectly fit. He looked in her ears, her eyes, felt her glands, sounded her heart, scaled her teeth, looked at her feet and examined her skin. Then, after asking Mrs Perry a few questions, he filled all the information into the booklet provided by the Guide Dogs' Association and handed it back to her.

'She's in fine fettle,' he said. 'I've entered it all into her dossier, signed it and now you can send the counterfoil back.'

The harness on again, Mrs Perry took hold of the metal handle and Bess led her mistress to the door. As Maurice opened it he said, 'It's stopped snowing and the sun is shining. Spring has returned.'

Mrs Perry smiled. 'Well, I can't see it but, thanks to Bess, I can go out and feel it all round me. She's an absolute blessing.'

We were just about to leave the surgery when the telephone called us back. I stood waiting as Maurice answered it and saw him smiling to himself as he listened.

At last he said, 'Why, yes. It's a good idea. I'll see what I can do for you.'

Putting down the receiver he chuckled. 'That was the Convent. Reverend Mother has had what she calls an "inspiration" – another of her bright ideas. She wants to know if I can get hold of a couple of lambs to graze that large lawn at the back. She says it will save the nuns having to mow it every week and cheer up the old ladies at the same time.'

I smiled. The nuns, who ran a home for infirm old ladies, were always full of schemes to make life pleasant for their charges. 'They won't like it much when the lambs get too big and have to go to market later on,' I said.

'Reverend Mother will think of something else by then. I rather suspect the lambs will end up in the deep freeze. She's a very practical woman.' He paused, 'Now where can I get— oh yes! Harry Wilkins up at Hillbrow Farm. He's bound to have some orphans. I'll give him a ring.'

A few minutes later he put down the receiver. 'The answer is "yes" and when I told him the lambs would be going to the old ladies' home he said Reverend Mother could have them for nothing. We'll pick them up when the weather is a little more settled.'

' "We"?'

'Well, you'd like to see the nuns again, wouldn't you? Two lambs in the car won't be any trouble and the sisters will help to cheer you up.'

I looked down at the miraculously resurrected dog on the floor, remembered our courageous blind friend who counted her blessings, and thought of the pleasure the old ladies in the home would have when they watched the lambs frisking on the lawn.

'I'm cheered up already,' I said.

Chapter Twelve

One thing about being a vet's wife is that you are very seldom bored. The animals you see and the people you meet fill your days with interest and variety and the unexpected happenings that occur keep you constantly on your toes.

Sometimes I hear the young, gathered round my kitchen table devouring doughnuts and coffee with their friends, complain about the 'tedium' of their lives and occasionally I comment, with what must seem to them nauseating complacency, that I, personally, wouldn't mind a bit of boredom every now and then.

I was reflecting on this one morning when Maurice was out on his calls and the telephone rang just as I was about to fill the washing machine. I called to John, who was home nursing a heavy cold, to take the message but, a few seconds later, he came into the kitchen.

'It's Pop. He wants to speak to you.'

Maurice's voice was full of urgency. 'I've got a pony over here stuck in icy water in a ditch about ten feet deep. He's only just been discovered by men working along the road and they're helping me to get him out. I need that sling in the store room. Will you bring it along right away? It's rather heavy but John can help you get it into the car.'

He gave me directions for finding the place and, putting down the receiver, I cast a rueful glance at my pile of washing and called, once more, to John.

The sling, very old and hardly ever used, was a strip of canvas and leather about six feet long and three feet wide, with metal bars on each end and a cast-iron yoke to hook on to the bars.

With the sling in the boot of my car, I set off at speed, ignoring John's protests at not being allowed to accompany me. Fifteen minutes later I pulled up beside a group of men and stared aghast at the sight of the pony wedged down in the ditch. Almost covered in muddy water, only his head, drooped in despair, and part of his back could be seen. Although I could tell from the churned-up banks on either side of him that he had been struggling violently, he seemed now to have given up the fight.

'How long has he been there?' I asked, as Maurice came up to the car.

'No one knows. At least a couple of hours.' He went round to the back and began pulling out the sling and I joined him as he laid it on the grass to straighten it out. Then he added, 'A passer-by with a dog found him and told these men who are laying pipes farther down the lane. They're digging away now at the sides of the ditch in order to make enough room to get the belly band underneath him. He belongs to a Mrs Barnes – she's over there.'

I followed his glance and saw the pony's owner, her hands clasped tightly together and her eyes fixed on the unfortunate animal. She turned as I approached and looked at me tearfully.

'How do you suppose it happened?' I asked.

She shook her head. 'We can only guess. He was in our field at the back of that wood. He must have jumped the fence and wandered over here. Oh dear! Listen to him – he's groaning.'

The pony, seeming at last to recognise that the men working on either side of him were coming to his aid, was uttering heart-rending cries of distress and Mrs Barnes' face turned white.

I tried to comfort her. 'He'll soon be out. Try not to worry. He'll probably be all right. At least he hasn't completely collapsed,' I said optimistically and then wondered whether I was looking too much on the bright side.

'I feel so guilty,' said Mrs Barnes. 'We only bought him yesterday, and as he'd been out all the winter in Kent, I thought he'd settle down better if I put him straight into the field. He's a present for our daughter Jane who's coming out of hospital next week. She's got to have lots of fresh air and exercise and the doctor said a pony would help her regain her strength. We've told her all about him and she was so happy but now—' She reached for her handkerchief and wiped her eyes. Then, seeing Maurice coming towards us she pulled herself together.

'Did you bring along the things I suggested?' he asked, and she nodded and pointed to a car and trailer.

'Masses of sacking and straw and I've put the lamp on in the stable.'

'Good. Well, the men have made it a bit easier now so let's hope he doesn't struggle because we've got to get this sling under him as evenly as possible.'

He took off his jacket and pulled on a pair of waist-high waders. Then he and one of the men carried the sling down to the slippery bank. To begin with, it seemed to go smoothly. Standing in the water, Maurice took a rope attached to the sling and pushed it under the pony and the man on the opposite side caught the end and began to pull. Then, suddenly, he slipped, called out in alarm and the poor animal, frantic with fear, began to struggle wildly.

'Stop! It's getting twisted.' Maurice reached down into the mud to recover his part of the sling. 'Wait a bit until he calms down. We'll have to begin again.'

Soon the pony, having exhausted himself, stood still and Mrs Barnes whispered fearfully, 'He'll go right down soon and then it will be all over for him.'

I said nothing but watched anxiously, my eyes fixed on Maurice, covered in mud and almost wet through, as he bent forward and pushed the rope once more under the pony. Then thankfully I saw the sling come out evenly on the other side, held firmly by the other man. The yoke was hooked over the pony's back and Maurice clambered up the bank.

'We won't need a block and tackle,' he said. 'There's a crane down the lane. He can be hoisted on to that.'

Ten minutes later the limp and seemingly half dead pony was pulled out of what was so nearly his watery grave, and lowered gently down on to the trailer. There was no time for congratulations. The men returned to their work, Maurice rubbed himself down roughly with a towel, then, lowering the back of the trailer, he and Mrs Barnes climbed in and began attending to the pony.

As they rubbed him down with sacking and wisped him with straw to stimulate the circulation I went to the car to get the heart and respiratory injection ready and, when that was in, Maurice opened the pony's mouth and poured down a stimulant drink.

'There you are, old chap,' he said. 'Now let's get you into that nice warm stable.'

As soon as we arrived in the yard of Mrs Barnes' house she let down the back of the trailer and looked at Maurice in dismay. 'My husband's not here and there's no one else about. How on earth can we get him out of the trailer on our own?'

'We're not going to be defeated by a little thing like that,' said Maurice grimly. 'A rope and a halter is all we need and a mighty big push from all of us.'

Stimulated by the injection and obviously longing for his stable, the pony rose unsteadily to his feet and aided by our combined efforts he struggled down the ramp and through the open door where he collapsed onto the straw.

This time I helped with the rubbing down while Mrs Barnes prepared a hot bran mash but, when it was offered to him, he showed no interest.

Maurice looked at his watch. 'I can't give him another injection for two hours and I've got some more calls to do. But first I must go home, have a bath and change. Stay with him, keep up the rubbing and try him occasionally with the mash. Let's hope he gets up before I return.'

A few minutes later we were speeding home and, as soon as we arrived, I poured out a good measure of whisky for Maurice.

'You have one as well,' he said, 'you've earned it too.' The telephone rang an hour later and Mrs Barnes said, 'He's been on his feet for a little while but he's breathing rather badly.'

'I've just got two calls to do,' said Maurice, 'then I'll be with you.' He picked up his case. I waved him goodbye and went to run a bath for myself.

Relaxed and warm I thought of the work I had planned to do that day and decided it didn't matter. There was always tomorrow and, if I had been able to help Maurice, it was well worth it. I just hoped the pony would recover and that the girl coming out of hospital would not have her homecoming saddened.

At tea time Maurice reported that, although the pony's temperature was below normal and he was still suffering from shock, he had taken a little hot mash. After the evening surgery he went back once and, when he returned, he looked pleased.

'His temperature is up a bit now but it's not very high. With a bit of luck he'll be OK. Already he looks very different from that half dead animal you saw this morning.'

'Well, you're the one who's half dead now,' I said. 'Don't go to sleep in that armchair. You should be in bed. You've had an awful day.'

He stared at me. 'Awful? Oh! I wouldn't say that. A bit unusual perhaps but very satisfactory.' He gave a huge yawn and stretched himself. 'One thing about being a vet – you never know what you'll be called upon to do. It all helps to make life interesting.'

I laughed.

'That goes for a vet's wife too,' I said.

Chapter Thirteen

It was the morning for collecting the lambs for the Convent and, having had a good deal of experience of travelling in Maurice's car with all kinds of animals, I felt rather apprehensive. Still, I comforted myself, two little lambs wouldn't be much trouble, so, dressed in practical clothes and armed with some old sacks, I was soon ready.

The farmer grinned as he lifted the two protesting lambs into the car. 'If I know anything about women,' he chuckled, 'these little fellows will never go into the deep freeze. They'll be petted and fussed over until they become real problems. Women are so muddle-headed where animals are concerned. Anyhow, tell the nuns that, if they can't cope with them after a while, I'll take them back. I'll fetch them myself.'

'Oh good!' I said, looking at the scrambling, bleating little creatures, 'because I draw the line at travelling with two fully grown sheep.'

I got into the back of the car, sat between the lambs and tried to hold them apart. They set up such a din that we could hardly hear ourselves speak.

'Got your wife well-trained, haven't you?' shouted the farmer approvingly as Maurice turned on the engine and gave a thumbs up sign as we drove away.

'Well-trained, indeed!' I snorted, with an arm round each woolly head, and Maurice laughed. 'It's all in a good cause. Think of the old ladies' pleasure, think of the sisters who have had to mow that big lawn.'

A hard little head butted against my shoulder and the other lamb began scrambling across my knees and, suddenly, with the farmer's remarks about women still ringing in my ears, I began to feel slightly victimised. I was, I decided, living in a male chauvinist world.

'Why is it,' I enquired rather acidly, 'that men think they are the only ones who can drive cars and that women should always look after the babies?'

Maurice chuckled. 'Can't you cope with them? Oh well! We'll change places if you like.'

He pulled into the side of the road and thankfully I took over the wheel. 'Perhaps they'll be calmer with you,' I said, and before letting in the clutch, I turned to look at him.

To my amusement I saw that he had put a thumb into each lamb's mouth and he grinned at me as they snuggled up against him, sucking away contentedly.

'You see,' he said smugly. 'My magic touch.'

As soon as we arrived at the Convent the door opened and a nun came down the steps to greet us. Beaming with pleasure and crooning over the lambs she led us round to the back where Sister Clare, who looked after the gardens, was waiting for us.

'We've put wire netting all round this part.' She indicated a vast expanse of lawn. 'They won't be able to get out and we've made a little gate here so that we can go in.'

Maurice put the lambs down and bleating loudly they began to frisk around, overjoyed at their freedom. 'They'll soon settle down,' he said. 'See they're beginning to nibble the grass already – but they'll need some supplementary feed for a while. A bottle of milk morning and evening should be enough.'

He gave a few more instructions and then we turned as Reverend Mother approached with her usual retinue of nuns, followed by a dozen or so old ladies positively twittering with excitement.

Reverend Mother smiled benignly. 'See how pleased they are. It's another interest for them. We're very grateful to you for bringing us these delightful little creatures.'

'Mr Wilkins says he will take them back when they get big and troublesome if you don't want to—' Maurice hesitated, 'well send them to market.'

Reverend Mother looked round at the Sisters questioningly and suddenly Maurice's meaning dawned on them.

'Have them killed?' A young nun looked up in horror, 'Oh! Surely not. We couldn't.'

'It's the logical end for animals bred for food,' said Reverend Mother calmly, 'but when the time comes I'll put it to the vote.'

The nuns sighed with relief and Maurice smiled. 'It's one of those situations we none of us like to face,' he said.

Invited to share their coffee break, we chatted with the old ladies and I watched admiringly as the Sisters waited on them, attending to the needs of those in wheelchairs and dealing patiently with some of the crotchety ones. It must be very depressing work at times, I felt, yet the nuns, many of whom were quite young, were among the happiest people we knew.

Our coffee finished we were about to leave when Reverend Mother drew Maurice aside. 'I wonder if you could help me, Mr Bowring. Since Mr Wilkins has been kind enough to give us these two lambs, I really do think they should end up in our deep freeze. Food is very expensive and we try to give our old ladies the best we can afford within our limited means. However, I can see I am going to be up against great disapproval.' Her eyes twinkled, 'Can you think of a way for me to get round the situation without upsetting the more sentimental members of our Community?'

Maurice nodded understandingly. 'Oh, yes. That will be quite easy to arrange. When the lambs become too big this lawn will no longer be large enough to give them sufficient grazing. So Mr Wilkins can then take them away, ostensibly to join his flock. Some time later you will receive a gift of deep frozen joints of lamb from a well-wisher who is a great admirer of your good work here. How's that?'

Reverend Mother smiled appreciatively and turned to me. 'Your husband is more than just our vet. He is one of our benefactors. He has taught us how to keep bees, he charges no fees for treating our animals, and now he is teaching me the art of diplomacy.'

Maurice looked highly embarrassed but was saved from replying by the arrival of Sister Clare.

'Oh Mr Bowring! I nearly forgot in all the excitement – it's our nanny goat. Will you have a look at her? I noticed yesterday that she wasn't chewing the cud and I think she's got a temperature. She's due to kid in a week's time.'

We followed her to a block of outhouses and Sister Clare pointed, 'There she is – peering out over the door. Isn't she lovely?'

She certainly was. All white, clean and sweet smelling, her yellowy intelligent eyes seemed to light up at the sight of her keeper and, rearing herself up on her hind legs, she laid her head gently on Sister Clare's shoulder. The nun stroked her lovingly.

'Poor Isabel. Never mind, you'll soon be better now that your doctor has come.'

Maurice took out his thermometer and the nun turned to me. 'She's such an affectionate creature. When I take her outside she follows me like a dog. Of course, I can't leave her to roam just anywhere or she'd eat all the vegetables and flowers; but I take her for a good walk around and then I tether her on that bit of rough ground over there and she thoroughly enjoys eating the brambles.'

Maurice withdrew the thermometer. 'Yes, it's certainly high. I'll give her an injection now and another one tomorrow. We must get her fit in time to kid.'

'We're hoping it will be twins,' said Sister Clare. 'In any case, we like having the milk. Lots of the old ladies enjoy it in their tea.'

I shuddered. 'Ugh! I certainly wouldn't! But I suppose you give them the choice, don't you?'

She looked at me in amusement. 'Of course! Do you think we stand over them threatening eternal punishment if they don't do as they're told? But seriously, once you acquire the taste – it's rather strong with a nutty sort of flavour – you find you want to go on drinking cup after cup. It makes lovely yoghurt too.'

Isabel, released now from Maurice's examination, bleated gently and settled down in the straw, her eyes fixed reflectively on Sister Clare. I thought what a peaceful scene it was: the young, hard-working nun, dedicated to serving humanity and the gentle, docile creature giving her love in return for the tender care she received. It all seemed very far removed from the world outside.

Maurice looked at his watch. 'We must be off. I have another call to make and it won't be as pleasant as this one. In fact, I think it will probably end up with a row.'

'Oh dear!' Sister Clare looked concerned. Then she smiled. 'Well, now, I'll say a little prayer for you while I'm doing the gardening and I'm sure it will all come out all right in the end.'

We laughed and waved goodbye and, as we drove away, I turned to Maurice. 'You make it sound quite alarming,' I told him. 'Where are we going for this confrontation?'

'Well, perhaps I exaggerated a bit but I've got to see that man who bought old Rampling's farm. Remember the rather truculent girl who brought her horse down when Sheila was spending the day with us? He's her father. Knows nothing about farming and won't take advice from me about his animals. He's just done a very stupid thing. Turfed out all the Friesians he bought with the farm, taken on a herd of Jerseys and says he's going to leave them out all winter to "toughen them up". Now, you can't do that with Jerseys when you're on high exposed ground like Hill Farm. They're very delicate little creatures and can't stand up to rigours of climate. He'll have casualties galore. His latest thing is pigs. Goodness knows how he'll treat them. If I were you, I'd stay in the car. Get immersed in a book. We'll probably have an up and down and that won't be very pleasant for you.'

I looked with interest at the tall, very smartly dressed man standing in the farmyard. To my relief, when Maurice introduced him, he merely gave a curt 'How do you do?' and stood waiting until Maurice was out of the car.

'You must see my sows,' he said. 'I've bought three in-pig gilts and one has farrowed already. I paid a bit over the odds for them, in fact I think I paid far too much but I'll see that I make up for it when I sell their litters. These country yobs won't catch me twice.'

Certainly a disagreeable man, I decided, and settled down to read the letters in the *Veterinary Record.* Half an hour later Maurice returned to the car alone. His face was flushed and he looked extremely angry.

'I'll talk about it in a minute,' he said as he drove quickly out of the yard and turned into the lane. Then he switched off the engine.

'I've told him he can find another vet to do his work. He's more than I can stomach.'

'What went wrong?'

'Well, first of all, he's put those pigs in the worst possible place. A very windy, cold spot with practically no sun. I told him they wouldn't thrive there but he refused to move them. He said he didn't believe in fussing over animals. The sow that has farrowed was scouring badly and the piglets didn't look too good either so I asked him to get help for me to inject her. He looked at me scornfully and said he wouldn't have thought a vet would be afraid of a pig. I explained what recently farrowed sows are like and repeated my request for a man to help me with a bit of plank or something but he said his pigman had gone to lunch. I rather think his men go early nowadays and don't hurry back. He won't keep them long anyway. So I suggested he should help me himself but he looked down at his beautiful tweed suit and said he wasn't dressed for it and, anyhow, he was paying me to do his work. I was getting a bit mad by then but the sow had to be seen to so I managed on my own somehow and came out undamaged.' Maurice paused and looked ruefully down at his trousers, 'Well, almost undamaged – she tore these a bit. Then, rather tactlessly perhaps, I told him he ought to get in touch with our friend Bill Boyd who would gladly give him advice on how to keep pigs properly. And that was when he flared up. Said he didn't need advice and wasn't going to have any yokels telling him what to do. So I said I would be sending in my account immediately and would be glad if he would find another vet to do his work.'

'How did he take it?'

'He didn't say a word. Just stamped off. He'll never be a farmer. I'll bet he sells up within a year.'

Maurice pulled the self-starter and, as we moved away he declared, 'That's one of the advantages of being in practice on my own. At least I can refuse to work for a man I dislike.'

I said nothing and Maurice grinned. 'I know what you're thinking. Not a very lucrative morning. First the Convent and now this.'

'Well, yes. And I don't like you losing a client.'

'Don't be so mercenary. What's more I haven't lost him – I've given him up. I don't want clients like that.'

We were having lunch when the telephone rang and Maurice went to answer it. He came back wearing a dazed expression.

'You'll never believe this. That was our friend up at Hill Farm apologising for his attitude this morning. Apparently he told his daughter all about it and she said I was right and he was wrong. She said he would lose his animals if he didn't follow my advice, so he's asked me to continue doing his work. He's going to move the pigs to a more suitable position and will bring in the Jerseys during the winter. What do you know about that?' Then he added hastily, 'Don't tell me. I know what you're going to say – women are much more sensible than men.'

I nodded. 'And a bit more businesslike too. Or would you call it "mercenary"?'

Chapter Fourteen

Maurice came into the room just as I had finished talking on the telephone.

'That was Bill Boyd,' I said. 'He wants you to call and Mary would like me over there as well.'

'She needs a good old feminine gossip,' said Maurice. 'Listening to Bill talking about pigs all day long must get a bit wearing.'

'I doubt it. She's still as a crazy about them as Bill is. She's like me, there. Utterly absorbed in her husband's work.'

'Very good thing too,' said Maurice and went to pick up his case.

As he opened the door of his car he saw me looking doubtfully at the passenger seat and, hastily grabbing a duster, he gave it a rub.

'OK now?'

I got in rather gingerly. 'Honestly – when I see other people's cars—'

'I know. You wonder why you ever married a vet.'

I laughed. 'Oh! well! It's worth it.'

'At least I'm not obsessed with pigs. I thought Bill's addiction might fade a little now that he's married, but not a bit of it. He still thinks they are the most fascinating creatures and I agree with him when he says they are highly intelligent though I think he overrates them a bit.' He chuckled. 'It's lucky for him that Mary is a pig-fancier too.'

I smiled as I recalled the time when Bill, a bachelor farm manager, had told us about the elegant girl he had met at a party. He had fallen in love at first sight but decided she would never want to share his life. When, however, at our suggestion, he invited her down to meet us he had discovered to his joy that her father was also a pig farmer and that she was as hooked on the creatures as he was.

Maurice broke into my thoughts. 'I expect Bill wants me to look at Hermione – that sow with the bad back. She probably needs another injection. I can't understand why she isn't better by now. It's a very odd business.'

I was just going to ask for more details when we turned into the drive leading to the farm and Bill, cheerful and hearty as ever, with Mary, his beautiful wife, came out to greet us.

'A drink first,' said Bill, leading us into the kitchen and then, as he filled the glasses he added, 'I want you to have a look at Hermione.'

'She ought to be OK by now, after all my treatment,' said Maurice. 'I can't understand why she has taken so long to respond.'

To our surprise, Bill roared with laughter and Mary's eyes were filled with merriment. We waited patiently for enlightenment while Bill took a large gulp of beer then, slapping the glass down on to the table, 'You'll be pleased to hear that the problem is solved,' he said. 'You'll never believe this and we only discovered it by chance ourselves but Hermione has been fooling us. She—'

'Wait a minute,' I interrupted hastily. 'Maurice hasn't told me about this. What is the story?'

He picked up his glass again and gazed into it, grinning broadly. 'Well, I thought I knew all there was to know about pigs but—' he paused and shook his head in wonderment, 'that's the beauty of it. They're the most intriguing creatures.'

He sat deep in thought, obviously reflecting with pleasure on the unique characteristics of his favourite animals and I glanced in amusement at Maurice who was looking extremely puzzled, and Mary smiling fondly at her big soft-hearted husband.

At last, with a slow chuckle, Bill looked up. 'Some time ago Hermione injured her back. The boar was a bit rough and she slipped and couldn't get up. She was out in the paddock at the time so we left her there as the weather

94

seemed settled and Maurice gave her a course of injections. She was pretty bad – well, you know how we fuss – so we fed her by hand and, of course, she got thoroughly spoiled, getting the best titbits and being treated like a duchess. We were very anxious about her – she's a fine sow. Then, two days ago, we had that night of heavy rain and Mary was worried about the poor creature lying out in the open so I went out to see if I could rig up some sort of shelter.'

He threw back his head and roared again.

'The artful old devil! She wasn't there. She'd got up and walked into her sty.'

Mary beamed at us and took up the story. 'The best part is that, next morning, she was out there again in the same place looking all pathetic and waiting for the usual goodies. Just to see what she would do, we gave her some and then tried to make her get to her feet. But, Oh no! She groaned and grunted as if to say "My poor back! I simply can't move," and she sank down again and looked hopefully at the apples I still had in my hand. We thought you'd like to see her putting on her act so we've left her there and we've kept on feeding her. But we've checked secretly. She goes into her sty every night and nips out first thing in the morning.' She rose from the table, 'Come and see for yourselves.'

'I've always said that pigs were highly intelligent,' said Bill. 'Now perhaps you'll agree with me.'

Sure enough, Hermione lay basking in the sunshine and looked up expectantly as we approached. But, as Maurice walked towards her, she grunted protestingly as if to say, 'Not another injection, surely? I'm no better for all your treatment.'

'You old fraud!' He addressed her in stern tones. 'I was really worried about you. Well, you're not getting away with it any longer.' He turned to Bill, 'Let's make her get up. I'd like to make sure she's really OK.'

'It'll take some doing,' Bill said. 'She thinks she's got us fooled. She's very clever.'

'Not as clever as we are.' Maurice turned away. 'I'll get Robert out of the car – he'll soon have her on her feet.'

He was back in a few minutes with Robert walking

quietly to heel, then, as they came into the paddock, he said, 'Go on boy. Fetch her!' and Robert bounded towards the recumbent sow. But as he drew closer he stopped in astonishment, slightly unnerved at the sight of the great creature glaring at him, and glanced back at his master.

'Go on,' Maurice urged, 'fetch her out,' and the dog began running round her, barking excitedly.

Alarmed and on the defensive, Hermione forgot she was an invalid, heaved herself up and made quickly for the safety of her sty with Robert close on her heels.

'Nothing wrong with her,' said Maurice. 'You're right, Bill. She's been shamming all this time. You'd better keep her in for a few days so as to get her out of the habit of lying there and being waited on.' He grinned. 'Well, you learn something new every day – that's the first time I've seen a play-acting pig. Any more problems?'

Bill shook his head. 'Nothing you can solve – at least, I don't think so. All the same, perhaps you'd better have a look at Phoebe – she's behaving very strangely at the moment. Keeps breaking out.'

'Well, pigs do, don't they? Not that yours have any reason to with that paddock at the back of their sties and all the cosseting they get. But there's no accounting for their whims.'

Bill disagreed. 'There's always a reason for their actions. I just can't discover Phoebe's motive.'

He led us into the piggery and pointed to a massive sow who grunted with pleasure at his approach. 'I've kept her in this morning although I don't like doing it but, as soon as I let her outside, she rushes to the fence, pushes her snout under the pig wire, heaves it up and runs riot in that allotment over there. She digs up the artichokes that are still in the ground and eats as if she hadn't been fed for a week.' He paused and frowned. 'She seems to have gone mad on them. It's no joke. The allotment holder is getting very awkward and beginning to throw things at her. Do you know, I've even got hold of some artichokes and put them in her feeding trough but she still goes on digging them up.'

Maurice laughed. 'Perhaps she's suffering from pregnant longings. When is her litter due?'

'In a fortnight.'

'It could be a mineral and vitamin deficiency. I'll give her an injection. Then you'll just have to keep her in until she farrows.'

When that was done Bill said fondly, 'All different characters, aren't they? Lovely creatures.'

Maurice grinned wickedly, 'You're right. They're fine animals. And there's nothing to beat a nice piece of pork. A ham sandwich always goes down well, too.'

Bill shuddered. 'No need to go into that. As a matter of fact, neither Mary nor I ever touch pork. It would seem like eating our friends.'

Maurice chuckled. 'Oh, by the way, there's a client of mine who has begun keeping pigs and has a lot to learn. He would appreciate some advice from you.'

It was while they were talking that Mary drew me aside and gave me some news that delighted me. On the way home, I passed it on to Maurice.

'It's early days yet,' I said, 'but Mary thinks she is going to have a baby.'

Maurice grinned. 'Well, that should take Bill's mind off his pigs for a bit.' Then he began to laugh and I looked at him questioningly.

'I was just thinking of Phoebe,' he said. 'You know – her "pregnant longings".'

I stared at him. 'What on earth—?'

'Well, suppose – just suppose – Mary also developed a craving.'

'For artichokes?'

'No.' A huge grin spread over his face. 'For pork.'

Chapter Fifteen

From time to time Maurice brings home small gifts that he has received from clients. Most of them are greeted with pleasure at the kindness of people who like to express their gratitude in this way but, occasionally – and I hasten to add, only very occasionally – he hands me something that causes me to stare at him in dismay. After the first stunned inspection I usually say, 'Well, it's the thought that counts,' and follow that up with 'but what on earth can I do with it?'

When the children were small it was comparatively easy to dispose of things like highly coloured, grossly inaccurate models of animals, photographs of dressed-up dogs and solid looking ponies, but they have long since outgrown that happy, uncritical age. Now, with their bedrooms hung with posters – fast sports cars and pop music groups on John's walls and literary posters and French Impressionists on Margaret's – they have very decided tastes of their own and are no longer grateful recipients of any old junk I try to unload on them.

Over the years we have received several peculiar gifts. There was the unbelievably hideous home-made 'antique' ironwork fire screen that worried me for a long time. As I didn't like to give it to our local jumble sale in case it should be recognised, and was unable to induce friends and relations to succumb to its charms, it was shunted around from room to room until it ended up in a shed where it turned so rusty that I was able to put it out for garbage with a clear conscience. There was a terrible oil painting that lived in the spare room until guests complained it was giving them nightmares and one or two other 'objets d'art' that made me wonder whether I was an ignorant Philistine or a super-cilious highbrow.

And now there was this. A tall, heavily decorated Victorian flower vase that I knew instantly would clash with every colour scheme in the house. I wandered round, placing it here and there, shaking my head and hating myself for being so ungrateful. Back in the living room, I was searching for a dark corner when the phone rang. Hastily dumping it on the television where it looked horribly incongruous, I picked up the receiver.

I listened carefully, wrote down the message and promised to pass it on immediately. Then I studied the list of farms where Maurice was working on this particular morning. Judging from the time, he should now be at Beech Farm, doing some pregnancy diagnoses. He had told me not to put anything through to him unless it was urgent as he had a full morning's work, but a cow that appeared to have broken her aitch-bone after a bad calving could not be ignored. I picked up the receiver once more. To my dismay, there was no dialling tone. I waited and tried again. Nothing. The line was out of order. I could make no outgoing calls although other people could get through to me.

I decided there was only one thing for it. Hurriedly backing my car out of the garage, I set out for the nearest telephone box. When I had reported the trouble, stressing the urgent need for quick attention, I rang Beech Farm. My luck was out again because there was no reply, so, abandoning thoughts of housework, I set out to deliver the message personally.

As soon as I drove into the yard I breathed a sigh of relief. Maurice's car, with Robert inside, was standing against the wall. A quick word with the dog and then I walked over to the farm buildings where, judging from the sound of men's voices and the occasional bursts of laughter, the pregnancy tests were still going on.

They didn't see me at first so I stood for a few minutes watching them at work. About ten cows were standing in a row and Maurice, well protected in his waterproof overalls, was examining a large Friesian. The herdsman stood by with a list waiting to write down the result of his findings when, suddenly, the cow lashed out with her hind leg. I gasped as Maurice dodged just in time and the men turned at my exclamation and stared at me in surprise. Then the herdsman's face broke into a large grin and Maurice came forward, holding his arm stiffly away from his side.

I gave the message and explained about the phone and Maurice said, 'I've nearly finished here. Only two more to do. Why don't you come along as well, now that you're out? You may find it interesting.'

I hesitated. A cow with a suspected broken aitch-bone wouldn't be a pretty sight but, as always, when it came to a choice between housework and watching Maurice dealing with animals, the animals invariably won. I withdrew to a safe position and waited.

It was a never-ending source of interest to me to observe the way in which he had to adapt to different patients and different conditions of work. Here, with large creatures contented and well looked after, the atmosphere was relaxed. Jokes – probably not quite so ripe now that I stood listening – were mingled with serious comments, sudden shouts to a cow to behave herself and sighs of satisfaction when the job was done. Farms, on the whole, were happy places and it was not surprising that Maurice liked his large animal work. Though it wasn't easy. Occasionally he has found himself lying on the ground in a muddy field, knocked down by an uncontrollable bullock; and he often came home bruised and sore after a tussle with a reluctant patient.

This was the rough, tough side of veterinary work. In contrast, I recalled the gentle way in which he dealt with small animals. Farmers, in general, are fond of their charges but the relationship between household pets and their owners is another matter altogether. To heal a sick dog or cat and bring joy to a young household or old people is a reward in itself. It was, as Maurice often said, a great life, and I reflected, not for the first time, how lucky I was to have a husband completely happy in his dedicated career.

The last cow done, Maurice came outside and I watched as he washed his arms and hands. Finally, picking up the bucket, he poured it over his chest, cleansing down his overalls at the same time. With a farewell joke from the herdsman we got into our respective cars and I followed Maurice out of the yard.

But there was no joviality at the next farm. 'When did she calve?' asked Maurice, gazing down at the South Devon, lying in the straw with her legs tucked under her, looking, as far as I could see, quite normal.

'Early this morning,' said the farmer despondently, pointing to the calf lying nearby. 'He's very big. We had a difficult job getting him out. Had to use a lot of force. Now she can't get up. She's tried several times but she never makes it. If it is her aitch-bone she'll have to go the knackers.'

'Well, let's see,' said Maurice. 'We may have to be a bit rough.'

He gave the cow a hard slap on her rump. 'Come on, old girl, get up! Get up!'

She began to struggle to her feet and, just as she was about to flop down again, the farmer gave her an even bigger thump and this time she managed it. But she stood with her hind legs wide apart rather like an ill-made toy. Then, with a protesting grunt, she sank down again.

'Well, that's not a broken aitch-bone,' said Maurice. 'If it were there would have been an awful cracking of bones grating together and she wouldn't have been able to stand at all. She's been badly knocked about, though. The nerves coming out from her pelvis have been terribly bruised and some of them aren't working properly. It will take about a week to ten days before she's right again.'

He looked down at the calf lying nearby.

'He can't get up either,' said the farmer.

'He's certainly had a rough passage,' said Maurice. 'Look at his swollen head and puffy eyes. And his shoulders are badly bruised by being forced through the pelvis. You'll have to milk the cow out and feed him from a bottle. It's essential that he should get the colostrum. He'll probably get up in a couple of days, but, until then, you'll have to turn him over several times a day.'

He opened his case. 'I'll give them both an injection to help get rid of the bruising and we'll see how they are in the morning.'

A few more words of advice and Mr Lawson began to look considerably happier. Then he said, 'I wonder if, before you go, you'd have a look at the wife's budgie? She thinks it's broken a leg. She's more upset about it than she is about the cow.'

Mrs Lawson was standing by the bird's cage looking very worried but she cheered up as soon as she saw Maurice. 'Oh! I'm so glad to see you, Mr Bowring. Poor Josephine got her foot caught up in the cage and dragged it out to get free. Now she can't stand on it. Do you think it's broken?'

Maurice opened the door of the cage and took out the little bird. He put his thumb under her beak to stop her pecking him and, with his other hand, he manipulated the leg.

'It's not broken,' he said at last. 'She's just twisted and wrenched it.'

Mr Lawson laughed, 'It's all good news today though this case is the least important.'

'All my patients are important,' said Maurice, and taking a pair of nail clippers from his pocket, he added, 'I'll just cut her claws. They're very long. That's why she caught her foot in the wire. Nature will heal that leg in about a couple of weeks.'

A few minutes later we were on our way home and, as I put my car away, Maurice drew up behind me. 'Good lord!' He pointed to the end of the drive. 'The telephone van is following us. That's service, if you like.'

The work was soon done, Maurice got out the glasses and the young engineer sipped his drink appreciatively. Suddenly, he caught sight of the vase on the television and, putting down his glass, he went up to it and stared hard. Then he turned to me, 'Lovely, isn't it? It caught my eye immediately because my wife and I have just moved into our first house and Betty has got the lounge done out in just those colours. Orange and blue. It looks really posh.'

Maurice coughed gently and looked pointedly at me, and I beamed at the young man. It took a certain amount of persuasion. Convinced that he ought not to accept the vase but obviously longing to present it to his wife, he demurred for a long time. Eventually, however, after I had shown him how it clashed with our colour schemes, he allowed me to wrap it up and went away, thanking us profusely.

Maurice smiled as he shut the door. 'You've probably given away a valuable antique but, at least, it's gone to a good home.'

At tea-time that day he came back from his afternoon calls grinning even more broadly and, taking an envelope from his pocket, he placed it on the table.

'No.' He shook his head as I reached out. 'Let me tell you the story first. I had to go to see a cat belonging to a very old lady. She lives in one room and, when I went in, she said, "Pussy's disappeared. She's here somewhere but she must have sensed you were coming and she's hidden away." The room was absolutely chock-a-block with all her possessions and we had to search for quite a while. Eventually, I found the cat hiding under the bed among piles of cardboard boxes and suitcases and dealt with her successfully. It was only a case of mites in its ears and I couldn't take any money from the old girl as she was obviously in what they call "reduced circumstances". Not to be outdone however, she went searching for something and then slipped this envelope into my pocket.'

He handed it over and, full of curiosity, I opened it, stared for a moment then burst out laughing.

'Two jelly babies!' I said.

'Well, come on – share and share alike –' said Maurice, and reaching out, he took one and popped it into his mouth.

'There you are,' he said, 'a very acceptable gift from another grateful client.'

Chapter Sixteen

'It's my morning at the Zoo,' said Maurice, 'would you like to come? We'll have a look at that lion cub and see how he's getting on in his new surroundings.'

'You mean the one that was brought into the surgery a few weeks ago?'

'Yes. George has put him in with some other ones of about the same age. Far better for him than being kept as a pet.'

I settled myself in the car and, as we drove away, I thought back to a morning when a man had come in with a lion cub pulling on a heavy chain. Smiling proudly at our astonished faces, he said,

'Grand little fellow, isn't he? Only twelve weeks old and tough as they come.

I was captivated at once and bent down to stroke him. The soft tawny cub coat still had its dark spots and the thick little legs with huge padded paws seemed out of all proportion to the weight of the small body. As I petted him, carefully avoiding his sharp claws, his owner turned to Maurice.

'I got him through an advertisement in the newspaper. My little girl is thrilled and simply adores him but he's a bit rough when he gets excited. He'll be safer for her to play with when you've dealt with him.'

I looked up in surprise and Maurice asked, 'What do you mean by "dealt with him"?'

'Well, when you've filed down his teeth and taken out his claws.' Picking up the cub by the scruff, the man held him out to Maurice. 'The people from whom I bought him said this was the thing to do.'

'They did, did they?' Maurice's face was grim as he

rubbed the struggling little animal under the chin. 'And how long will you keep him? Nine months? A year?'

'Oh, when he gets too big for us he'll have to go into a zoo. But we'll give him a good time while he's little and then, of course, he'll want to be with his own kind. We'll visit him regularly, though. We're great animal lovers, as you can guess.'

Maurice nodded, put the cub on the floor, pulled up a chair for his client and sat down himself. 'I think,' he said evenly, 'that you have been misled. I wouldn't dream of mutilating a wild animal like that and I don't know any other vet who would do it either. You say you will give him to a zoo when he gets too big but with no claws he couldn't be put in with other lions – he'd have no means of self-defence and he'd be massacred. So he would have to be kept in solitary confinement. Even a female will lash out from time to time and no one is going to take the trouble to search for a mate who is so placid that she will never have a go at him. So he wouldn't have much of a life, would he? In fact, it would be very difficult to find a zoo – a good one, anyway – that would take him.'

The man looked bewildered. 'I never thought of it like that.' He paused, then, bending down, he pushed the cub away from his chair. 'Stop gnawing at that leg, you young devil.'

There was a tiny snarl, the cub's lips curled back and he stared up with angry eyes. His owner lifted him, still snarling, and held him tightly in his arms. Then he said helplessly, 'But what on earth am I to do with him? What do you advise?'

'He obviously can't play with your little daughter,' said Maurice, 'he's quite fierce already. And it won't be easy to get a zoo to take him. Most of them have enough cubs as it is. They're almost two a penny, but, if you like—'

'Two a penny? Good God! I paid a hundred pounds for him!'

There was a long silence. 'So I've been "done" have I?' The man stared down at the cub.

Maurice nodded, 'I'm afraid so. Unfortunately there are

lots of unscrupulous people about who are exploiting this fashion for exotic pets.'

The other man frowned, 'Exotic pets? Well, yes, I suppose you're right. One does rather like to cause a bit of a sensation with something out of the ordinary. Still – a hundred pounds up the spout – an expensive way to learn. But there it is. What do I do now?'

'If you like,' said Maurice slowly, 'I'll ask the Superintendent of our local Zoo whether he can fit this little fellow in with some cubs who have been reared on the bottle. They're roughly the same age and, after a bit of skirmishing, he would probably be accepted.'

And so it had turned out. George had agreed and the owner had sensibly taken the cub to his new home.

As soon as we arrived at the Zoo the Superintendent came towards us and peered into the back of our car. 'Hope you haven't brought any more "foundlings",' he grinned, 'that monkey has been quite a problem.'

I was puzzled. 'What monkey?'

'Didn't he tell you? Why, he said he'd have to take it home if we hadn't room and that you would go mad if he did, so—' George chuckled, 'not wanting to break up a happy marriage I gave in to his blackmail.'

I stared at Maurice and he smiled back, completely unabashed. 'Let me see – when was it? Oh, yes. Last week, when you went up to town with Margaret. I had a call to see a pet monkey. The people concerned had had it since it was a baby but it had grown so destructive that they'd had to put it into a room by itself. They told me they thought it was ill. When I got there I was horrified. The room was tiny and very cold and the poor little creature, bored and lonely, had torn off all the wallpaper and practically wrecked the place. It was certainly ill – it had pneumonia. I could have put it to sleep, in fact the owners themselves thought it would be a good idea, but it had had such a rotten life that I thought I would like to give it a chance of something better. So I twisted George's arm a bit and he – kind-hearted man that he is – agreed to take it over.'

'Thank you very much, George,' I said feelingly. 'You've

saved me from a fate worse than death. I've always rather drawn the line at taking a monkey into the home. How is he?'

'Much better. He's a different monkey altogether.'

'I suppose the problem now is how to get him to live with the others.'

'We can't put him in with a colony,' said George, 'but we'll find him a mate and see how he reacts. I expect he'll settle down eventually. Your other *protégé* - the lion cub - is doing well. The other cubs chased him round a bit but he held his own and now he's one of the family. I think he's going to be a fine fellow. Come and see him.'

I found it difficult to distinguish what I thought of as 'our cub' from about four others, rolling and playing together, but Maurice spotted him at once and smiled with satisfaction. 'Yes, he's a lovely little chap. Have his former owners been to see him?'

'They were here yesterday,' said George, 'very pleased with themselves for having donated him to the Zoo. Now, we mustn't waste any more time – I want you to look at the Yak's feet. I think they'll have to be done today.'

Maurice looked at him in astonishment. 'Do them now? With all these people around? I thought we were going to arrange it for an evening when the Zoo is closed.'

'Can't be done.' George shook his head. 'I've got to take some Guanacos over to Wales and then I have to go on to another zoo to collect an ostrich. After that a couple of keepers are going on holiday and we'll be a bit short-staffed. Anyway, come and have a look at him and see what you think.'

Out in a field, away from the main part of the Zoo, we came to a large paddock surrounded by heavy chain-link fencing. At the far end I saw a heavy, ugly animal grazing. He looked rather like an ox but with a long, shaggy, black coat hanging nearly to the ground. His hairy tail was like that of a horse, there was a slight hump along his back and his horns were thick and curved, ending in sharp points. With a white fringe hanging down his face and big mobile nostrils, he looked a very tough customer indeed. His legs were short and stumpy and I could see that his hard, horny feet were very overgrown.

Maurice watched him moving slowly over the grass and turned to George. 'You're right. They must be done now. The weight is pushing him back on to his heels and he's getting lame. I'll just get my hoof clippers from the car and then I'll load the dart gun.'

While he was gone, George went in search of other helpers and returned with two men. 'This is Bert,' he said, and I smiled at a young pleasant-faced man, 'and this is Dick.'

Dick was only a lad, with long hair and a cheerful grin which became even broader when George added, 'He's the one who's going to be used as bait. He can run faster than we can.'

I looked from him to the Yak, already growing restless as he realised something was going to happen, and said, 'Rather you than me. How are you going to set about it?'

'Line him up to where Mr Bowring is standing,' said Dick. 'It's a question of getting the dart in the right place. He's very truculent – chases anyone who dares to go into his territory.'

Maurice began loading the dart with the anaesthetic.

'I should think he weighs between eleven and twelve hundred pounds – I'd better give him—' he looked up as a group of spectators appeared in the distance. 'Oh lord! Now we'll have some crazy comments. Keep them at a distance, will you?'

Seeing that something interesting was going on, the group surged forward, children gazing round-eyed over their ice creams and the adults discussing the situation in loud voices.

'That man's got a gun!' A large blonde woman wearing tight white trousers pulled at her husband's arm. 'Oh gawd! they're going to kill that poor animal.' She advanced towards us, dragging her unwilling spouse along with her.

'You shouldn't do that in front of children. It's cruel and wicked.'

'It's all right, Madam.' George grinned. 'We're not going to hurt him. He's got to have his toe-nails cut and the vet is going to give him an anaesthetic so that he won't feel anything.'

'Well, I never!' She stared at him then said disbelievingly, 'Go on! You're pulling my leg. No one ever gets an anaesthetic just to have their toe-nails done.'

She muttered something to her husband who nodded and glared suspiciously at the dart gun and looked closely at George and the keepers who were conferring together.

'Right then,' said Dick, 'I'll go in now. Mind you leave the gate open for me to get out quickly.'

'Keep right back, please,' said George to the onlookers. 'Don't distract us – this animal is very dangerous.'

'I don't like it,' said the large lady. 'I can't bear to see animals getting hurt.'

Her concern evidently did not include the keeper and I felt myself growing angry. Maurice glanced at me in amusement.

'Don't get worked up. People always think we're sadistic torturers when our only aim is to help the animals.' He nodded to Dick who was still waiting for his signal, 'I'll stay here near the gate so try to get him within range.'

The lad took up a bucket and went to the entrance and, suddenly the group of spectators fell silent as he opened the gate and went in, holding out the bucket invitingly.

The Yak looked up, hesitated, and then as Dick still walked forward, he gave a great snort and pounded towards him. Ignoring his overgrown hooves he covered the ground at an incredible speed, making straight for Dick with his great head down, ready to use his terrible horns on the intruder. Dick turned and ran like mad, slamming shut the gate just in time as the furious animal charged at the chain-link.

Maurice stood waiting, gun at the ready, as the Yak charged again, and the fence seemed to bend under his onslaught. I glanced at the onlookers standing spellbound at this sudden transformation from an apparently placid animal into a wild, dangerous foe and then I looked at Maurice who was waiting for the Yak to calm down. Another charge and then, frustrated, he paused and stood still for a few moments. Right on cue, Maurice fired and the dart landed fair and square in the Yak's haunch.

110

There was a long 'Ooh!' from the spectators and the woman who had said she couldn't bear to watch pulled her husband towards the barrier, and stood horrified but fascinated as the Yak snorted and retreated— but only for a few yards. Then he turned, looked furiously at Maurice and pounded towards him. He stopped short of the chain-link, his huge grey nostrils distended and then, to my surprise, he began walking aimlessly around in large circles.

'They often do that,' said George, 'and sometimes they go a bit berserk and keep on charging until they fall down.'

This time, however, the Yak contented himself with moving round and round until gradually the circles grew smaller and smaller. Suddenly, he stood still. Long streams of mucus were coming from his nostrils and, with his tongue hanging out, he began to pant. Still fighting against the oblivion that was overwhelming him, he made a last great effort and began to charge but his legs gave way and he collapsed onto the ground. Snorting furiously, he tried to rise but rolled onto his back with his feet sticking up in the air, the great hooves still lashing out and his tail swishing wildly. But as his head rolled from side to side, the horns digging into the ground, I could see the fierce eyes clouding over at last.

'I think that's about it,' said Maurice. 'I don't want to give him any more anaesthetic. We'll just have to be very careful.'

Armed with a length of rope, George and the keepers opened the gate and went into the paddock, followed by Maurice carrying the heavy hoof clippers. Made of cast iron with cutting edges of steel, they weighed nearly five pounds and were about two feet long. As they approached, the Yak seemed to become aware of their presence but George quickly looped the rope round a waving back leg and he and Bert hung on to keep it still while Maurice began cutting the horny hoof, dodging back every now and then as, in spite of the men's efforts, the leg jerked towards him. Dick knelt down at the Yak's head, holding the horns and whisking away the flies that began gathering round the animal's eyes. He gently stroked the grey nose and I marvelled at the genuine affection these keepers had for all the creatures, lovable and unlovable, in their care.

Soon Maurice was working on the front feet and then, the job completed to his satisfaction, he stood back. At that very moment, as the men relaxed their hold on the rope, a leg shot out in his direction. I gasped in alarm but he was on the alert and, swinging aside, escaped injury.

A few minutes later, he injected the antidote and then they all came out of the paddock.

Dick grinned at me. 'I reckon that's cut down my chances of survival now, because when I go to put in the bales of hay, he's going to be quicker off the mark than ever.'

We stayed waiting to see the Yak recover consciousness but, the excitement over, the group of onlookers began to drift away. The blonde lady complained loudly that she thought it was all rather horrible and unnecessary.

George looked after her reflectively. 'It's funny the way folk react. Even when we're helping an animal to stay contented and healthy, they accuse us of being cruel.'

Maurice nodded. 'There's a great gulf between people who work with and for animals and those who have very little contact with them. Now—' he grinned, 'have you any more "cruel" jobs for me to do?'

George shook his head and laughed, once more his cheerful self, and Maurice added, 'Good. Because as soon as this fellow is on his feet, I must be on my way. I've got to see a parrot. It's off its food and plucking out its feathers. The old lady who owned it has died and her nephew thinks it's pining for her.'

'Oh! No!' George groaned in mock horror. 'Not another one for us, please. Anyhow, the parrot house is full.'

'Don't worry. The nephew is very fond of the bird and wants to make it happy. It's probably only moulting. Look—' he pointed, 'the Yak is coming round.'

Sure enough, he was beginning to roll over and soon he was swaying on his feet. Then, with a rather subdued snort, he looked round and ambled off to his shelter.

'He'll be grazing again in about an hour,' said Maurice. 'I'll look in on him again tomorrow but he should be OK.'

We said goodbye and, as we went on our way to the parrot, Maurice said suddenly, 'When I was looking at that lion cub I remembered what his owner had said about people liking to have pets that caused a bit of a sensation and it made me recall something else. Do you remember John and his lizards?'

'Why, yes, of course. That was a similar case, I suppose – our son revelling in the admiration of his friends because he had unusual pets. It's human nature, after all.'

Pulling up outside a house in a quiet road, Maurice took his case and went in to see the parrot. As I sat waiting for him, memories of John when he was about twelve years old kept me amused.

He had seen lizards on the moors in Devonshire and, from then on, he became obsessed with these elusive little creatures, searching for them on sunny heathland and bringing them home in plastic bags. He tried to keep them alive in an old tropical fish tank but, when it dawned on us what was happening, Maurice had taken a hand, insisting that if John wanted to keep them properly he must build a 'lizardry' in the garden. A large sunny rockery was selected, protected from marauding cats and birds by wire mesh, and there the lizards settled and lived happily. For a long time that corner of the garden was the joy of John's life. Even I, who never liked cold-blooded creatures, was fascinated and used to enjoy watching them as they darted in and out of their hiding places and sunned themselves on the rocks. John and Margaret would bring their friends in to admire them and sometimes, showing off their knowledge of the facts of life, would announce that one or other of the females was pregnant. I had my doubts but, to my surprise, they were proved right because, on several occasions, tiny little creatures about half an inch in size appeared and gradually grew to adulthood. They all hibernated in holes in the rocks during the winter months and it was a great day in the spring when John announced that the lizards were out in the sun again.

Then I remembered how, with growing ambition, John went too far and came home one day showing with enormous pride, his latest catch. I had been very alarmed.

'A snake! John! It's an adder!'

'Of course it isn't,' he said scornfully. 'Do you think I don't know the difference? It's a harmless grass snake.' He showed it to his father. 'Isn't he beautiful?'

Maurice nodded, 'Yes, he is beautiful. But you can't keep him. You'd better go and put him back where you found him. He can't go in with the lizards – he'd eat them – and, taken from the wild like this, he would have to be given live food. Are you prepared to feed him live frogs?'

I shuddered and Margaret, almost in tears, said, 'Live frogs! Oh! John, you couldn't!'

Our son's face was downcast as he gazed with longing at the snake, its greeny-brown skin glowing in the sunshine. Then he looked at his father.

'Well, let me try feeding him dead things. Or pieces of meat. If I put them on a string and wiggled them about, he might think they were alive.'

Maurice shook his head. 'You won't fool him like that. Besides, you'll have to put him in a container – that old tank again. Not much of a life, is it?'

Convinced at last, John reluctantly returned the snake. Accompanied by his sister, he made a sad pilgrimage to the place where he had found it, put it down on the grass, half hoping, he told me afterwards, that it would refuse to leave him, but when he saw the lightning speed at which it slithered off to its familiar haunts, he came back an ardent new convert to the conservation of wild life in its natural habitat.

The lizards stayed on for a year: then other interests took over and, one day, John gathered up all the inhabitants of the rockery and set them free.

I was still dreaming of the past when Maurice came out of the house. As he settled himself in the car, he said, 'I was right about the moulting but the owner was right too when he said he thought the bird had been pining for the old lady. Parrots are funny creatures. They live a long time and get very set in their ways. If the person who looks after them dies, then they are quite lost. Everything is different and they do pine. What's more, they like the opposite sex in humans to themselves. This particular one is a male and had been the old lady's pet for many years. The nephew took it into his house while the wife was away staying with friends and, although he tried to get friendly with the parrot he had no success at all. It screamed at him constantly and tried to peck him – wouldn't let him get near. But now his wife has returned and the bird has taken to her in a big way. Holds its head up to be rubbed, makes ingratiating noises and is quite happy again. He'll be OK now. All the same—'

I read his thoughts. 'I know. I agree with you. I hate to see birds in cages. Even those vultures at the Zoo.'

'Talking of vultures,' said Maurice, 'I feel rather like one myself. Let's get home to lunch. Bread and cheese and beer, I think, don't you?'

We were just finishing our snack meal when we heard a car coming up the drive and Maurice looked out of the window.

'Ah! It's Mr Mead. I expect he's brought some more cats to be "done".'

He went outside, took two cat baskets from a middle-aged man and stayed talking for a few minutes. Then, after putting the cats in the surgery to await their operations, he returned to the kitchen.

Watching the car disappearing down the drive, he said, 'That man and his wife are a marvellous couple. They devote their spare time to looking after old people's cats, getting them "doctored" when necessary and seeing that they get veterinary attention when they're ill. They collect the cats, use their own petrol to bring them down here, and very often, if the owners are poor, help out with the fee.' He paused and then added thoughtfully, 'Now, they are what I call *real* animal lovers.'

Chapter Seventeen

Concern for animals, however genuine, can be overdone, and sometimes situations arise in which there is conflict between the vet and the owner. Veterinary surgeons, on the whole, are not regarded with the same awe or given the unquestioning trust that people accord to their doctors. This, as Maurice often says, is probably a good thing and keeps the vets on their toes, but there are times when a strongly held belief that animal treatment is only a second-rate form of medicine can be rather exasperating.

We came up against this attitude one morning when a tall, anxious-looking man, holding a young Alsatian bitch on a lead, stood scrutinising the consulting room. He was already late in arriving. Patients for operations have to be brought in early so that the tranquilliser has time to work before the anaesthetic is given but, instead of apologising, he said, rather brusquely,

'I want to watch Mr Bowring doing this operation.'

With my mind on the waiting room already full of clients and with Maurice busy talking on the telephone, I asked quickly.

'Have you any particular reason?'

He hesitated, and I waited, rather regretting my question. I should have told him straight away that Maurice always refuses any such request. To have an owner watching him is distracting and a hindrance to concentration.

At last he said, 'Well, yes. You see, I'd like to make sure that Betsy won't be roughly treated in order to make her unconscious.'

Speechless for a moment, I stared at him. Then I said, 'Do

117

you think we are going to hit her over the head with a spade
or something like that?'

'No. Of course not. But I'd like to be here in case anything
goes wrong.'

Wondering what possible use he thought he could be in an
emergency, I was relieved to see Maurice putting on his
overall.

'You'd better ask Mr Bowring,' I said, and went to look in
the waiting room which seemed, at the moment, to be
unusually noisy.

All the chairs were occupied by clients with cat baskets on
their laps or dogs lying at their feet and all eyes were gazing
at a youth who stood near the door. He was holding a cage
containing a Mynah bird and, suddenly, I realised what the
commotion was all about. Hopping up and down on his
perch, the bird was spreading alarm and despondency among
the dogs by giving a most realistic impression of a warlike
cat. Hissing, snarling and emitting long drawn out miaows,
he had them all in a high state of tension. The youth was
gazing blandly at the ceiling, obviously enjoying the sensation
he was causing and, suddenly, at one particularly malevolent
wail from the bird, there came a series of yaps from a little
terrier and the other dogs began to growl ominously.

'It's all very well,' grumbled a fat lady, holding a poodle
tightly by the lead. 'He's upset my Roland. He'll get
over-excited – it's bad for him.'

I walked over towards the youth and, at that moment, the
bird put his face close to the bars of the cage, and said in a
gruff masculine voice 'Where's that bloody cat? Come on in
puss, puss, puss.' There was a brief pause, then, very clearly
and distinctly, he poured out a string of words that, to put it
mildly, are not usual in polite circles.

The fat lady's mouth fell open in horror, an elderly
gentleman put down his magazine and looked at the bird over
the top of his spectacles, and two small boys turned almost
purple in their efforts to suppress their mirth.

The youth grinned at me disarmingly, 'Sorry about that,'
he said. 'Dinah doesn't mean anything, she only imitates
what she hears at home. My Dad's got a bit of a temper.'

I gazed at the bird in amusement, then, seeing that she was about to show off her vocabulary once more, I said hastily, 'I think you'd better come in first,' and led him in to see Maurice.

To my surprise, the tall man was still there, standing beside his dog, and Maurice was in the office searching among his papers. I went in and closed the door and when, at last, he found what he was seeking, I asked, 'Why are you letting that man stay? I thought you hated people watching operations?'

'He's very tenacious, isn't he? But don't worry – I'll get rid of him all right.'

Going back into the consulting-room, he said, 'Mr Richmond, I'd be glad if you would wait outside while I see my other patients. That's if you really want to stay. I shan't be operating for another hour.'

'Oh, very well.' Bending down, the man began to undo the dog's lead which was attached to a hook in the wall, but Maurice said,

'You must leave her here. I want her kept calm.'

Reluctantly he went outside and the youth came forward, holding out the cage.

'She just needs her claws clipping.' He jerked his head towards the door and grinned. 'I came in last and got in here first. Dinah was upsetting them a bit out there.'

Maurice smiled and, taking his clippers, he opened the cage door. Immediately, Dinah, who for the last few minutes had remained quiet and subdued, let out a flow of language that would have done credit to the proverbial trooper.

'Phew!' said Maurice. 'That's a nice way to greet your doctor! Another one who doesn't trust me!'

Holding the bird in his left hand, he dealt swiftly with the overgrown claws and, as he put her back into the cage, he said, 'Next time you come in you'd better keep her covered. Some of my more refined clients might take offence at her eloquence.'

As the youth went out of the room I said, 'Conversation must be a bit colourful in that household.'

119

Maurice grinned, 'Colourful certainly, but rather limited I should think. Now, let's have the next problem.'

An old lady came in slowly, carrying a bundle in a shawl. She looked at us suspiciously for a moment then, gradually unwinding it, she placed a dog on the table.

I stared at it, horrified. The poor little mongrel was quite unable to stand. He was terribly emaciated and the smell coming from his mouth made me feel sick. Drawing back involuntarily, I glanced quickly at Maurice. His eyes were full of pity as he looked gravely at the wretched creature and then he gently stroked the dog's sunken back.

He looked up and asked quietly, 'How old is he? About fourteen?'

The old lady nodded, glaring at him fiercely.

Maurice passed his hand quickly in front of the dog's eyes. 'He's practically blind as well.'

She nodded again and Maurice waited patiently. At last she said, 'I want you to give me some medicine to make him better.'

He stared for a moment then slowly and compassionately shook his head.

'I'm afraid there's no medicine for his condition — extreme old age. There's nothing I can give you that will make him young again. But you know, don't you, that he's very unhappy? His life has become a burden to him. Will you let me put him to sleep? It's the kindest thing you can do for him now.'

She glared at him again, in total disbelief.

'I want some medicine and some ointment for his eyes.'

There was a long, agonised silence. The sad little heap on the table never stirred and I grew hot and angry inside at the cruelty that went under the name of love.

'Please, believe me,' said Maurice at last. 'If I could help your old friend, I would. And it really is wrong to keep him in this state.'

Suddenly the woman reached out, picked up the pathetic bundle and wrapped him in the shawl.

'You're just a murderer!' Her voice was shrill and hysteri-

120

cal. 'I don't want him killed. When he's meant to go he'll go. You're a vet   you ought to try to make him better.'

'I can't. Don't you see?' Maurice's eyes were growing angry but he still spoke pityingly.

'I know you love him dearly but you must put him first. Don't let him go on suffering.'

She shook her head violently.

'He's not suffering and I don't believe in killing.'

She went towards the door and Maurice followed her.

'Don't go yet,' he said pleading, 'sit down in the waiting room for a while and think over what I've said.'

He held open the door and stood watching for a moment then he came back.

'She's sitting down, anyhow,' he said. 'Let's hope she'll come round to the right way of looking at things.'

Ten minutes later, when I went into the waiting room, I saw her sitting in a corner, talking to an elderly man who was holding a cat basket. I spoke for a minute to another client and while she was giving me some details, I heard the man say, 'It's the end of the road for my old Timmy, I'm afraid.'

The old lady muttered something and the man shook his head and said bluntly,

'Well, I'd rather be dead than like your poor dog.' She put her handkerchief to her eyes and he added, 'Selfish, that's what you are.'

'Where's the next patient?' Maurice opened the door and I ushered in the client to whom I had been talking.

Ten minutes later, the elderly man came in with his cat and, after giving his old friend a quiet word of farewell, he looked up at Maurice.

'It's a very hard thing to say goodbye like this.' His eyes were moist and he turned away for a moment. Then as he went to the door he said, 'I've persuaded the lady out there to change her mind about her poor old dog. I should get her in quickly if I were you.'

I followed him out and he stopped by the old lady. Bending down he said something softly and she nodded shakily then, her face grey and drawn, she handed me the bundle in the shawl.

'Would you like to come in and see how peacefully he will go to sleep?' I asked gently, but she shook her head and, as her tears began to fall, the old man put his arm round her shoulders.

'Come and have a cup of tea with me,' he said. 'I know how you feel.'

The remaining cases went smoothly and quickly and then, as I escorted the last client back through the waiting room where Mr Richmond still sat patiently, I saw a schoolboy sitting in the corner holding a puppy. For a moment I didn't recognise him then I exclaimed,

'Andrew! What a pleasant surprise!'

He beamed as he held out the puppy for my inspection and I found it difficult to believe he was the frantic youngster we had tried to comfort a few weeks ago.

'What a lovely little Springer Spaniel,' I said. 'Is he yours?'

He nodded happily then his smile faded and he said,

'Mummy said we ought to take Mr Bowring's advice. I didn't want to at first but—' he looked down at the puppy, 'I can't help loving him. He's not Barry, of course, but he's awfully nice.'

'What have you called him?' I stroked the silky little body and the puppy wriggled ecstatically and nearly jumped out of Andrew's arms.

'I haven't got a name for him yet. I thought I'd ask Mr Bowring.'

'Come along in,' I said, 'I expect you want him immunised.'

Maurice was delighted. 'Well, you've certainly got a fine little fellow there.' He took the puppy and examined him closely, 'couldn't have chosen better myself. My favourite breed.'

Andrew watched as the injection was prepared and, as Maurice took hold of the puppy, he asked anxiously, 'Will it hurt much?'

122

'Hardly more than a pin-prick. He may give a little yelp. But this stuff has saved millions of dogs' lives so it's worth it.'

The boy looked closely at the syringe. 'I wanted to bring him to you because I'd like to see what you do. I've decided to become a vet myself.'

The puppy never even uttered a squeak as the needle went in and, as Maurice rubbed the place to disperse the injection, he said,

'You've paid me a great compliment although I wasn't able to save Barry. I should think you would make a very good vet. You'll have to work hard at school to get all those high grades in the sciences but, if you really put your mind to it, I've no doubt you'll succeed. Would you like to come out with me sometimes on my rounds so that you can see what it's all about?'

Andrew's face lit up with joy. 'Could I really? I promise I won't be a nuisance.'

'Of course you won't. Give me a ring when you break up for the holidays and we'll fix things up.'

He was just going out of the door when he turned and came back. 'I nearly forgot. Can you suggest a good name for my new puppy?'

For a moment Maurice pondered then, glancing down at the little dog's coat – liver-coloured with a faint tinge of auburn – he said slowly,

'The best dog I ever had was a Springer Spaniel called Robin. I've never called another one that because I loved him too much to be able to repeat it. But I'll give the name to you.'

'Robin—' Andrew tried it out, then bent his head down to the puppy, 'You're going to be called Robin. It's a lovely name.'

As he went away, Mr Richmond stood up.

'At last!' he said. 'I was wondering if you were ever going to get around to operating on my dog,' and, following me into the room, he planted himself at the head of the operating table.

Maurice eyed him disapprovingly, 'Do you mind standing farther away, please – you'll be in my way there.'

I frowned as a signal to Maurice and said,

'Just a moment. I want to ask you something.' He followed me into the office and shut the door. 'For heaven's sake!' I exclaimed, 'Why are you letting that man stay? He's going to be a menace while you're operating.'

He laughed. 'I'll talk him out of it. Want to bet?'

I looked at him doubtfully, 'He's a very obstinate type. Why didn't you tell him to go in the first place?'

'He was pretty insulting with his hints of brutal treatment so I thought I'd like to teach him a lesson. I'll bet you a pound he'll leave before the first incision.'

'Done!' I said. 'A pound.'

'Not that I'll ever get it,' said Maurice.

Betsy growled softly as he lifted her on to the table and immediately Mr Richmond said,

'She can sense she's going to be hurt.'

I glared at him but Maurice remained silent and, taking a piece of cotton tape, he tied it round the dog's muzzle.

'Here — why are you doing that? She doesn't bite. It's quite unnecessary and she doesn't like it.'

His eyes glinting but his voice well under control, Maurice explained patiently, 'One never knows how a dog will react when a needle is put into the vein. Sometimes the gentlest animals will turn on you. It's only for a minute — I take it off as soon as the anaesthetic begins to work.'

'I don't—' began Mr Richmond but Maurice stopped him.

'Do you want me to operate on your bitch or would you rather go elsewhere?'

The man subsided and, trying to ignore his presence, I drew out the dog's front paw and Maurice fixed on the tourniquet above the elbow joint to bring up the vein. Usually, when I am holding an animal I talk to it soothingly but the critical spectator made me self-conscious. We worked in silence and uneasily I wondered whether Maurice had forgotten his bet. If this wretched man remained to question everything he did, it would be most unpleasant.

In a short time Betsy began to go limp and I untied the tape and took it off her nose. As she slumped farther down under the influence of the anaesthetic, Maurice opened her mouth and tested the reflexes of tongue and jaws. After that, he tried a hindleg, a foreleg and finally the eyes.

'Right,' he said, pulling out the needle, 'she's had enough. Now let's get her on her back.'

When she was attached by each leg to the table I pulled out her tongue and let it hang from one side of the mouth then I went to fetch the instruments in the steriliser.

Once more Mr Richmond approached the table.

'Is she still breathing?' he asked nervously and then, as I pointed to the chest rising and falling, he gave a sigh of relief but remained standing close to Maurice, watching as he began to shave the area of abdomen where the skin incision had to be made.

Picking up the scalpel, Maurice began to talk.

'Now I'm going to cut her open from here to here.' He pointed to an area about six inches long, 'and then all the intestines will be exposed. I shall put forceps on to all the arteries that have to be cut, pull out the uterus and tie off and remove the ovaries. It won't be a pretty sight, I warn you. I think you should put on a white overall as you are standing so near – you might get blood on your clothes. At the same time, I might as well make use of you, so you can keep an eye on Betsy's breathing and let me know if you think it's getting feeble.' He paused. 'Before I begin I must make absolutely sure you really want to watch. I've had people passing out at the sight of blood and I don't want you to distract me by crashing on the floor. I'm afraid, if you do, I shall have to leave you there.'

I went to get a white overall, noticing as I did so that Mr Richmond had gone quite pale. But he nodded as Maurice looked at him questioningly and I decided I'd have to watch him as well as his dog.

Poising the scalpel immediately over the mid-line of the abdomen, Maurice said,

'Right.'

Then, in the split second before he began to make the incision, Mr Richmond gave a great gulp, muttered something and rushed to the door.

'Do you think he'll be all right? Ought I to go and look?' I asked anxiously, but Maurice chuckled, 'Plenty of chairs in there. He can put his head between his knees. Let him be. Just thank goodness he's gone.'

I listened for a moment but there was no heavy thud and, looking extremely pleased with himself, Maurice began to operate.

When he had nearly finished and he was suturing up the wound, he looked up at me and grinned.

'You owe me a pound. It was a dead cert with a blustering type like that. A verbal picture of an operation is nearly always enough to put most people off.'

When Betsy was lying comfortably under her blanket I opened the door and, rather shamefacedly, Mr Richmond came in and went over to look at his dog.

'She's in fine shape,' said Maurice. 'You'll be able to take her home this evening. By the way, are you all right now?'

'All right? Oh, I see what you mean.' Mr Richmond's self-confidence made a rapid comeback, 'You're mistaken. There wasn't anything wrong with me. I'm not the squeamish type. But I decided at the last minute that I was really in the way. Didn't want to hinder the good work, you know.'

Shutting the door behind him, I said, 'I'll bet he tells his friends he watched the operation from beginning to end. You described everything so well that he'll get away with it.'

'Probably – and bore everyone to death.' Maurice took off his overall and heaved a great sigh.

'What a surgery! I've been sworn at, accused of being a murderer and suspected of sadism. I think I'd better warn young Andrew what he's in for if he persists in wanting to be a vet.'

Chapter Eighteen

We seemed to be in the midst of a period of night calls. Three times in the last week Maurice had had to turn out to go to urgent cases.

'I think,' I said rather crossly, when in the middle of our first deep sleep, we were awakened for the fourth time by a demanding voice, 'that you ought to train your clients better. A whelping bitch could surely wait till the morning.'

'In the ordinary way, yes. And I do tell them what to do in advance but, if things get difficult, it's perfectly reasonable to call me out. This is a new client, though. I'm not sure I've ever been to the house.' He looked at the address on the message pad. 'I don't recall that name, do you?'

I looked at his scribble. 'Can't read it. Still, the address is clear.'

'He had just gone down the drive and I was dozing off again when the telephone rang once more.

'Mrs Dicker here. I rang a short time ago. Are you the vet's wife? Well, there's no need for him to call now. My own vet has arrived.'

My mind began to boggle. 'Your own vet? Do you mean that you rang two at the same time?'

'Yes. I was so worried about this whelping. I just couldn't remember what I had been told to do. You know how panicky one gets. I rang my own vet first but I thought I'd better be on the safe side, so I got on to one or two more.'

'One or two?' I could hardly believe my ears.

'Yes, and I must stop the other one coming so I'd better ring off. I don't want three vets' bills.'

Well, you'll jolly soon get them all the same, I thought. Then I asked,

'Do you ring several doctors if you think you need one in the middle of the night?'

'Oh, no. That's different. You have to stick to the same doctor but it doesn't matter with vets, does it?'

'It certainly does—' I began indignantly, but she rang off and I was left muttering to myself. I picked up a book to calm myself down but I was still awake when Maurice returned.

'She rang to put you off just after you'd left,' I said. 'Of all the nerve – you must have been furious.'

He shrugged his shoulders resignedly.

'Stupid woman! She was obviously out of her wits with panic but there was no point in letting fly. Peter Rallton was there too. He'd just got back from a bad calving and looked worn out so he expressed himself pretty forcibly. She won't do it again, anyway – not when she gets our bills.'

After four disturbed nights Maurice was rather tired next morning and, unfortunately, surgery was extremely busy. The hot weather was bringing in the patients with a vengeance. Dogs seemed to be the main casualties. There were fat ones with heart troubles, others with skin irritations caused by the owners giving the same amount of food as they did in winter, lots of dogs with fleas and puppies needing inoculations. When the last client had gone Maurice studied the list of messages that had been coming in since breakfast time.

'Lord knows when I'll be finished today. Never mind, I'll have a really early night to make up for lost sleep.'

'Oh, dear!' I looked at him in dismay. 'We're supposed to be going to the theatre. I expect you've forgotten because I booked up ages ago. It's that play we all wanted to see and Wednesday was the only evening I could get seats.'

There was a long silence, then I said,

'You're too tired to go, aren't you?'

He nodded ruefully. 'Do you mind very much?'

'No, of course not.' I knew that if I showed my disappointment he would force himself to go. 'I expect John or

Margaret will be able to rustle up a friend to take your place.'

He relaxed. 'That's fine. I'll make it up to you another time.'

The play was very good and we enjoyed every moment but, what with dropping off the other girl at her home, we didn't get back till well after midnight. Maurice's car was in the garage and the house was quiet. I breathed a sigh of relief and hoped the spate of night calls had abated.

When John and Margaret had gone upstairs, I lingered in the kitchen for a while, drinking tea and turning over the pages of a magazine, knowing full well that I was reverting to bad habits. I am, unfortunately a 'night' person, never wanting to go to bed at a reasonable hour and never wanting to get up in the morning, but Maurice is the opposite, yawning at ten o'clock in the evening and able to enjoy the dawn. Over the years we have worked out a suitable compromise, both going to bed at what we each consider to be the wrong time. But when I have been out anywhere I find it impossible to relax and I give way to my 'owl-like' nature.

This evening I enjoyed my stolen time, alone except for Robert in his bed in the corner of the kitchen. Unusually for him, he had taken no notice of us when we came home but now he began to get restless. I turned to look at him and saw, to my dismay, that something was wrong. Holding his head on one side, he whimpered unhappily then began furiously scratching at his right ear and shaking his head violently. Suddenly he began running round and round the room, rubbing his ear on the floor and working himself into a complete state of panic. It was obvious that he had a grass seed in his ear and immediately my imagination took over. I thought of it going deeper and deeper inside with every movement of his head. Perhaps it would penetrate so far that he would need a general anaesthetic to dig it out. Suppose it couldn't be found? Suppose he died under the anaesthetic? Suppose— I knew I was being ridiculous but, without thinking any further, I ran upstairs for help.

Maurice lay sleeping deeply. Even switching on the light

didn't disturb him. I stood wondering what to do, my mind on the dog going frantic downstairs.

At last he stirred and opened his eyes. 'Hello – did you enjoy yourselves?'

Then he saw my face and shot up in bed. 'What's wrong? Have you had an accident?'

'It's Robert,' I said urgently. 'I think he's got a grass seed in his ear. You'll have to come and see what you can do.'

Without waiting for an answer I went downstairs again and, to my relief, he followed me into the kitchen.

'Well – I don't know!' He looked at me reproachfully, 'Did you really think I hadn't noticed it? I'm going to take it out tomorrow. I settled him down for the night, put some olive oil into the ear to soften the seed and gave him something to make him sleep.' He stared at the teapot and the open magazine. 'If you hadn't stayed up drinking tea with the light on, he would have slept till morning.'

Taking a bottle of olive oil, he made Robert go back into his bed and poured the liquid into the affected ear.

'Let's hope he goes to sleep again. We'll have to wait and see.'

Soothed and calmed down, Robert eventually settled and, before turning out the light, Maurice looked at me and grinned.

'Another silly woman calling me out of my bed in the middle of the night. And a vet's wife, at that!'

Chapter Nineteen

Returning from a visit to the Convent, Maurice gave me the latest news.

'Isabel, the goat, has had twins, the lambs are a great success and now Reverend Mother has come up with another scheme for combining business with entertainment for the old ladies. She's going to get a pig – an in-pig gilt, to be exact.'

I laughed. 'What a good idea. The old girls will love going down to the sty and scratching the pig's back with a stick. I'll come with you next time and see the new arrival.'

Later that week we went over to the Convent and found Sister Clare and another nun admiring their new charge. 'Reverend Mother has given me an assistant to help me with the extra work,' said Sister Clare. 'Sister Teresa is a farmer's daughter so she is in her element.'

We smiled at the young nun who seemed to be very pleased with her new job, admired the massive Large White busy devouring a heaped-up trough of food at great speed and with many satisfied grunts and snuffles, and soon we were joined by Reverend Mother.

'It was good of you to ask your friend Mr Boyd to give us the benefit of his expert advice,' she said to Maurice. 'He came yesterday evening, thoroughly approved of our arrangements and told us what to do when the piglets arrive. He has also promised us the services of his boar later on when she is ready for another litter. We're very lucky to have so many kind friends and benefactors.'

Maurice grinned, 'We're all laying up treasure for ourselves in Heaven,' he said. She smiled appreciatively and turned to me.

131

'Now, Mrs Bowring, perhaps you can help us out. We want a name for this delightful creature. Mr Boyd suggested Gertrude but I don't think that is quite suitable because we have a Sister Gertrude who is— well, shall we say, rather plump, and it might hurt her feelings. Have you any ideas for us?'

I pondered deeply. Various names passed through my mind but each one seemed as though it might be applicable to members of the Community. A pig in a Convent – it was a bit difficult. Then, suddenly, as I gazed at the big white animal, my memory went back to my schooldays in Belgium and I exclaimed,

'Why – of course! Blondine!' Then, translating hastily, I said, 'Blondie.'

The two Sisters giggled and Reverend Mother smiled approvingly, 'Most appropriate. We certainly have no Sisters bearing that name and, really, when you look at her, she couldn't be called anything else. But, tell me, why did you say "Blondine" at first?'

'It came out of the past,' I explained. 'I was at a Convent school in Belgium for six years and we had a Reverend Mother rather like you – very resourceful and businesslike—' I hesitated for a moment, wondering if I had gone a little too far, but Reverend Mother's eyes were twinkling, so I went on. 'She decided it would be a good investment to keep a pig, and a large white sow arrived, much to our delight. We christened her Blondine and I'd forgotten all about her till this very minute. She was a great character.'

'Mr Boyd says pigs are highly intelligent creatures though I find that hard to believe,' said Reverend Mother, looking at her new acquisition who, having demolished her enormous meal, was preparing to have an afternoon nap in a sunny corner of her enclosure. 'However, we shall be perfectly content if she just turns out to be a good mother.' Then, catching sight of my raised eyebrows, she added hastily, 'I don't, of course, mean that a good mother is not intelligent – Oh dear! What have I said?'

For once, Reverend Mother looked flustered and Maurice

and I burst out laughing. Wishing the nuns good luck with their new venture, we drove away, still chuckling.

On the way home, Maurice said, 'What was all that about a pig at your school in Belgium? It's the first I've heard about it.'

'It was all a very long time ago,' I said, and, as I began to tell him, I saw once more the Convent with its smooth lawns, formal flower-beds and ornamental pond; with the vegetable garden and the pleasantly untidy part round by the outhouses and the chicken runs.

I don't know who christened the pig when she arrived but the name stuck and 'la chère Blondine' became the fashion. We visited her regularly, scratched her back and fed her with apples or anything else we thought she would fancy. Not that she was fussy. She seemed to appreciate everything that came her way and she grew larger and larger and more and more friendly.

Towards the middle of term, she produced a litter of eight squealing, battling babies and her sty became a centre of pilgrimage for nuns and pupils alike.

All this adulation began to go to Blondine's head and, not content with receiving homage and tit-bits in her home, she decided to go in search of more.

She began breaking out, wandering all over the gardens, followed closely by her rollicking, destructive brood. However often she was shooed back to her sty, however strong the barriers erected, it made no difference to Blondine. She had developed itchy trotters and was determined to see the world.

In the process, the flower-beds were rooted up, the lawns round the pond became a sea of mud and Sister Gudule, the head gardener, said that in her opinion this was the Gadarene swine all over again and a clear case of devilish possession.

We pupils found it very amusing and did our best to encourage this delinquent behaviour. It was, in fact, whispered that one of the English girls – always more ingenious than the docile Belgians – had opened the sty gate in the first place, but of this there was no proof. Then, one hot afternoon, we were having lessons in the garden when she

133

lumbered right into our midst causing great hilarity and utter confusion. The sight of our exercise books being trampled and torn to pieces sent Sister Léonie, our form mistress, very nearly into hysterics and marked the beginning of Blondine's downfall.

The end came when she and her offspring got into the vegetable garden and left it in such a state that according to rumour Sister Gudule had delivered an ultimatum to Reverend Mother. Either Blondine must go or she, Sister Marie Gudule, would apply to the Holy Father for a dispensation from her vows.

Unlikely as this was, it made a good story and we were not really surprised when Reverend Mother decided to cut her losses.

One morning the sty stood empty and forlorn and we were told that Blondine and her rampageous progeny had been sold to a neighbouring farmer. We mourned for a few days, but suddenly examinations appeared like thunderclouds on the horizon and life became grimly studious.

A few weeks later, on one of the last days of term, we had black pudding for lunch. This was not, on the whole, a favourite dish with the English girls, especially as it was served, Belgian fashion, with stewed apricots. However, we were preparing to make the best of it, when a whisper went round and we looked down at our plates with horror.

It couldn't be – they wouldn't – not Blondine!

It was no use the nuns denying, pleading or even threatening – we just couldn't bring ourselves to eat that black pudding.

In the end we were given large slices of Dutch cheese and mashed potatoes which we ate with a great show of outraged virtue. No one ever discovered who sent the whisper down the tables, but it was obviously one of the English girls. The same one, probably, who helped Blondine to freedom by leaving open the door of her sty.

I came to the end of my story and back to the present as Maurice pulled up outside our house. He sat grinning to himself for a few moments, then he asked,

134

'The girl responsible for all the trouble – did they ever find out who it was?'

I shook my head and smiled reminiscently,

'No,' I said, 'I never owned up.'

Chapter Twenty

The call from the police came on Saturday when we were having lunch. As soon as the conversation was over Maurice picked up his case and began to check the contents.

'Let me see – needles, gut, antibiotic – yes, everything's here.' He turned as he went to the door. 'A nasty business up at Stewart's farm. He's had a pack of dogs chasing his sheep and one ewe is very badly bitten.'

Two hours later, when I was in the garden, I saw his car coming down the lane, and he looked grim when he joined me. 'That ewe was in an awful mess. Mr Stewart's man, the one who is part-time shepherd, came up with me to the fields above the farm and there she was, poor thing, looking more red than white. She was covered in blood. The shepherd thought I'd have to put her down but I managed to stitch her up though it was a difficult job. She was numb with shock, of course, so we got her on her back and I spent over an hour cutting her wool, putting antibiotic into each gash and stitching up. We had to turn her from side to side – there were bites all over her – you wouldn't believe ordinary dogs could be so savage. I put about sixty stitches in, gave her an injection and then we got her into a trailer and took her back to the farm. I thought that was that, but Mr Stewart told me that when he'd seen the sheep all huddled at the end of the field, he'd rushed up in his Land Rover with his gun and, although he was too late to get a shot at the dogs, he recognised one of them – the leader of the pack. He told the local police and they're coming down here in about half an hour.'

'They?'

'Mr Stewart, the dog, it's owner and a policeman.'

'What have you got to do? Put the dog down?'

'It's only a suspect so far. Mr Stewart said he had seen the dogs running around in a pack for some time. He knew where this one lived. I've got to see if this suspect has any sheep wool inside him. I can't help feeling sorry for the owner if he has, but, there you are – it's his fault for not keeping the animal under control. If Mr Stewart had managed to catch the dog in the act he could have shot it quite legally. That's what townspeople so often don't realise. They let their dogs run wild and, if they're not used to livestock, they begin chasing them just in fun. Then it suddenly becomes serious, the old hunting instinct comes to the fore and what was at first a game, becomes a massacre.'

'You say there was a pack of dogs chasing the sheep. Did one start them off?'

'Yes. There's always one who is the leader. Actually, a sheep could stand up to a dog if it wanted but it's too timid and it runs away. That makes the dogs chase them and then all the old savagery comes out. Of course, sheepdogs run after them when they're rounding them up but they're properly trained and the sheep know them.'

A quarter of an hour later, we stood in the surgery in a strange group. Mr Stewart, stocky, red-faced and grim, the dog's owner – a middle-aged man looking extremely angry – and a policeman who stood unmoved and silent by the door.

Handing his dog over to Maurice, the owner said, 'All this is quite unnecessary. My Rufus wouldn't hurt a kitten. He's the gentlest, friendliest dog I've ever had. Look at him.'

Rufus, a very handsome Labrador/Alsatian cross was trying to lick Maurice's face, wagging his tail and living up to his master's description.

'Can you imagine a dog like that savaging anything?' His owner turned to Mr Stewart. 'I've a damn good mind to sue you for personal inconvenience and humiliation.' Mr Stewart said nothing but it was plain from the expression on his face that he had no doubts at all about the identity of his sheep's attacker.

Maurice put on his overall and the owner looked at him in

alarm. 'What exactly are you going to do? You can't operate on him without my permission.'

'No, of course not. No question of that.' Maurice's voice was gentle. He obviously felt sympathy for the man but, having seen the suffering of the wounded ewe he had to keep an open mind. 'All I have to do is to make your dog sick. If there is no sheep's wool in his vomit then he's cleared of suspicion.'

He went to the cupboard and took out a jar.

'I'm going to push a small lump of washing soda down his throat. That will make him bring everything up almost immediately.'

Suddenly the atmosphere became tense. The policeman came up to the table, the owner stood as near to his dog as possible and Mr Stewart moved in behind him. Only the dog seemed happy, wagging his tail at everybody and trying to get down from the table.

I began to wish with all my heart that I hadn't come into the surgery. It had seemed the natural thing to do at the time but now I realised that it was probably a matter of life or death for this lovely animal whose fate depended on Maurice's next action. It was clear that no one wanted to see the dog proved guilty with the possible exception of the farmer. Although I hesitated for a moment as to whether or not I would stay, the drama of the situation held me and I watched as the owner held his dog's head steadily while Maurice opened the jar and selected a piece of soda about the size of a hazelnut.

With a swift movement he pushed it down the dog's throat saying, 'You'd better stand back. Here it comes.'

There was one great heave followed by two more, and Rufus ejected the contents of his stomach on to the surgery table.

I heard an incredulous gasp from the owner as Maurice took a pair of forceps and, picking out a lump from the vomit, held it out to the policeman and then to the dog's master.

'Matted sheep's wool,' he said.

There were several other lumps plain to be seen and many separate strands, enough to convict the dog twice over.

Maurice lifted Rufus down and let him stand beside his master who took out his handkerchief and wiped his forehead. He turned to the policeman, 'What does this mean for my dog?'

The constable cleared his throat. 'Well, sir, it's obvious, isn't it? The dog's guilty.'

I turned away, unable to look at the beautiful animal, guilty in our eyes yet, in reality, completely innocent. A creature who was only following his natural instinct and had no knowledge of right or wrong.

Then I heard the policeman say, 'If you don't agree to having him put down, the case will have to go to a magistrate's court and the evidence is dead against him. If he is put to sleep then you will only have to pay damages to the farmer – that will include the vet's bill for stitching up the ewe – and you will also have to pay her value if she dies.'

Mr Stewart spoke at last and even he sounded sympathetic. 'It could have been worse. You're lucky that the lambing season is over. You would have been held responsible for any abortions or dead lambs in the entire flock.'

'Of course I'll pay the damages,' the poor man said as he looked sorrowfully at his dog, lying quietly now on the floor. 'It's him I'm thinking about. Couldn't I sign something to the effect that I'll keep him properly under control in future?'

'It's for you to decide, sir. The vet can't put him to sleep without your permission at the moment. Later on, it would be another matter.'

'Once a sheep worrier, always a sheep worrier,' said the farmer.

I knew then I couldn't see it through. I looked across at Maurice to see if he wanted me to help in any way but he shook his head and jerked it towards the door. Thankfully, I slipped outside and went round into the house.

Ten minutes later the cars drove away and Maurice came quietly into the room and sat down in his armchair.

'I know what you're thinking,' he said.

'Well, it seems all wrong to me. You don't shoot a tiger at the Zoo if he attacks a keeper or another tiger.'

'This dog wasn't a wild animal. Domestic pets and

140

livestock have to be kept under control. It's the price they pay for their share of our civilisation. You wouldn't have thought it wrong if Mr Stewart had shot the dog when he was tearing at that ewe or if you'd had to stitch her up as I did. Rufus was a lovely animal in our company but he was a very different creature when he was leading a pack and it wouldn't have been long before he did it again.'

'Am I just being sentimental, then?'

'I'm afraid so. I was sorry when I put the dog to sleep – sorry for the owner, poor man. But the dog was perfectly happy up to the end. One injection that he barely felt. But his master – everybody was sorry for him. Now,' Maurice went out to the kitchen and put the kettle on to boil, 'what you need is what you're always doling out to other people – a cup of good strong tea.'

I felt better when I put down the empty cup.

'There's one thing I'd like to know,' I said. 'Mr Stewart said "once a sheep worrier, always a sheep worrier". Is that really so?'

'As a general rule, yes. Though I remember when I was a boy staying down at my friend's farm in Kent. They had a couple of young dogs who were showing signs of chasing the sheep and the old man put them in a field with a ram. Only for a short time however, because the ram put his head down and charged and the dogs had to run for their lives. They never ganged up on sheep again so it can sometimes be cured if they're young enough and it's taken in time.'

I picked up a book. 'I think I'll have a quiet read to calm me down.'

'Good idea. What's it about – animals?'

'No fear,' I said. 'I've had just about enough for one day. This is a nice clean murder story.'

Chapter Twenty-one

Uncontrolled dogs running loose are not the only problems farmers have to contend with. Townspeople out for their week-end walk in the country often do great harm, and although this is mostly caused by thoughtlessness, the trouble they leave behind is sometimes very serious. Gates are left open, crops trampled down and fences damaged by happy wanderers unwilling to keep to the footpaths.

We had an instance of this when, on Maurice's half day, we went to tea with friends of ours who had a small farm.

'I hate to talk shop on a social occasion,' said David when we were sitting in the garden admiring the view and enjoying Betty's home-made cakes, 'but I'm worried about that bullock you saw a couple of days ago. The one that was lying down right away from the others. He had a slight temperature and you gave him an injection. Well, he's no better – in fact, he's worse. He gets to his feet occasionally but he groans and I think he's in pain. Will you have another look at him?'

Betty glanced at me and I laughed. 'Yes, I'd like to have a walk. I need it after all those lovely cakes.'

Soon we were out in the field behind the house and David pointed, saying, 'See – there he is, lying down again beside the hedge.' As we approached the young black-and-white Friesian, he began to struggle to his feet then, groaning, he sank down again. We went up close to him and, instead of showing the usual wary curiosity of a grazing bullock, his brown, velvety eyes were dull and listless.

'Good lord!' Maurice exclaimed. 'He's gone down very suddenly. The antibiotic hasn't had any effect. It must be something more than a colic or a chill.' He paused, deep in thought. Then he looked at David. 'I rather suspect a foreign body.' Gazing round the field he stared for a moment at a stile at the far end. 'There's a footpath running through here, isn't there? Do you think he's picked up some litter left lying about?'

David shook his head. 'I'm very careful – walk the field every day. On the whole, people – local folk – are very good, though at this time of the year families often come by car, and sometimes they break through the wire in order to get to those woods over there in search of wild flowers. Oh! Wait a minute—' he turned to his wife. 'How long ago was it that we found those bits of broken wire on the ground?'

She thought for a moment. 'Almost two weeks. But we picked up all the bits – well, we thought we did. Surely that's too long ago to be the cause of any trouble?'

'No,' said Maurice, 'it's quite possible. Mind you, if this bullock had swallowed a bit of wire, it wouldn't necessarily cause trouble. Not unless it perforated the stomach or gut. Then it would let bacteria in and that could cause peritonitis.'

'But a hard thing like that,' I said, 'wouldn't the animal spit it out?'

'They're not like horses who pick everything over with their lips before they chew. Cattle, being ruminants, swallow without chewing.'

'Surely, though' – David was looking very worried – 'he would have shown signs of pain before this?'

'Not necessarily. Many animals don't show any symptoms until it's too late. And remember – cattle have four stomachs. The food goes first of all into the big one – the rumen – and when that's full, the animal regurgitates a mouthful at a time which it then chews thoroughly. Then it's swallowed again and goes down into the next stomach, and digestion begins there. If a foreign body, heavier than the food, has been taken in, it would sink down to the bottom of the rumen and wouldn't come up again into the mouth to be chewed. Even then, with a bit of luck, it might pass through but, if it has got lodged, it could penetrate the rumen and gradually work through to the heart. So you see, it can be quite a time before

144

any obvious symptoms show, and by then, it's usually too late. These are terminal symptoms, I'm afraid. Sunken eyes and going downhill fast.'

We stood in silence, gazing sorrowfully at the poor little bullock looking at us so mournfully, doomed to an early death on this lovely summer day.

'I'll get on to the knacker then,' said David at last.

Maurice nodded.

'The only thing to do. We can't let him go on suffering. I'll go over afterwards and do a post-mortem.'

'Oh, dear!' Betty turned away. 'It's no use – I'll never get used to things like this. I hate seeing them go to market but at least they've had a good life out here. To think of those horrible footpathers cutting the wires and scattering the bits around.'

It cast a shadow over the lovely afternoon and, when David had telephoned the knacker and arranged for him to pick up the bullock, we said goodbye.

On the way home a thought suddenly struck me. 'Couldn't you have operated on the poor little thing?'

Maurice shook his head regretfully, 'Not a practical proposition, I'm afraid. In the case of a very valuable cow I might have had a go but I'm sure it was too late for the bullock.'

An hour later he went off to the knackers and, when he returned he said, 'Yes, it was a piece of wire. Look –' he held out a strip about two inches long – 'it had pierced the pericardium. The poor little beast must have been in great pain.'

He went to the telephone and, when he had finished talking he came back and poured out a drink.

'David is furious,' he said, 'and quite rightly. He says it's not surprising farmers hate people wandering over their fields. They seem to think when there's a footpath it gives them freedom to roam everywhere.'

Two days later Betty rang me. 'David is still hopping mad,' she said, 'and the footpathers have done it again. Well, not the same thing but they left a lot of rubbish in the hedge

145

- plastic bags too. We're putting notices up all over the place and David says he's a good mind to put a bull in the field.'

'That's a bit drastic, isn't it?'

'Well, yes. In any case, it's against the law to put a bull into a field where there is a public footpath.'

Maurice laughed when he heard the news. 'He'd never get away with that. There'd soon be trouble.'

A fortnight after that he returned from visiting the farm saying, 'David has come up with a good idea. He's put up a notice that says "Please keep to the footpath and beware of bullocks." It's worked wonders, apparently. People go through the field very quickly and quite a few change their minds and go back.'

'But why should they be scared of bullocks?' I asked curiously.

'Well, lots of townspeople don't know or aren't quite sure about them. They tend to think they're young bulls. Oh, and by the way – he's put another notice up beside the woods. It says "Beware of snakes!" He chuckled and added, 'I must say, he has my sympathy.'

I thought of the pathetic little bullock with his sad eyes and untimely death.

'Mine too,' I said.

Chapter Twenty-two

'I have a bit of a problem this morning,' said Maurice, as we set out for the Zoo, 'a simple job really but it's complicated by the fact that the patient is an epilectic giraffe.'

'Is that Miranda – the one you were telling me about the other day?'

'Yes. We've been watching her for some time. She's a fully grown female and one half of her cloven hoof is growing over the other. It needs to be cut back to level it up as it's beginning to cause discomfort. Unfortunately, no anaesthetic can be given as, in the first place, we can't estimate her weight to the nearest half ton and secondly, she's exceedingly nervous and throws a fit if she gets the slightest bit agitated.'

'A giraffe in a fit!' I exclaimed. 'That must be a terrifying sight.'

'It's very dangerous for the animal. She throws herself around, bashing her head against the walls, and her legs go all over the place. There's always the fear that she will break her neck.'

'Has she always been epileptic?'

'No. She was bought from another zoo when she was quite young and the epilepsy developed when she became adult. I expect it's a case of inbreeding. That's one of the troubles nowadays. There are many animals that zoos can't import from their country of origin any more and, although there are zoos all over the world and animals are interchanged, enormous creatures like giraffes are very difficult to transport. Consequently, they tend to get inbred. It's happening to lots of captive animals.' He paused. 'A few days ago we tried to do Miranda's foot with a saw. George fed her apples,

147

which she loves, while I worked away down below but she soon noticed the vibration and we had to stop.'

George had obviously been working on the problem as well, for when we arrived at the Zoo, he said, 'I've come to the conclusion we can't do the job all in one go. But, if you could hold an axe over the toe and give it a sharp blow with a hammer, you might get a bit off or, at least, make an impression. Then, by doing this over a period of days, we could eventually cut it down. It won't be easy because we shall have to do it between the bars.'

'That sounds a good idea,' said Maurice. 'I'll have to be careful, though, not to cut the quick or she'll throw her usual fit.'

As we approached the giraffe enclosure we saw that Miranda was the only one outside and George said, 'We'll let the others out when we've finished. I want you to have a look at the young one. That trouble with his joints is getting worse, I'm afraid.' He paused. 'Damn! I've forgotten the apples – I'll just nip back and get some.'

He disappeared and Maurice and I stood watching Miranda. She was about fourteen feet tall and her large eyes and mobile ears seemed perpetually on the alert. I admired her beautiful fawn coat with its chestnut.

'Isn't she graceful?' I said, as she moved towards us.

Maurice nodded. 'That's the way she walks. Giraffes move their two left legs together, then their two right ones. It's quite peculiar. Both feet at one side off the ground at the same time.' Then he added, 'A giraffe has the most powerful kick in the animal world and, when they swing their neck, they can break open a man's skull with their head.'

'She seems very friendly all the same,' I said.

'Oh! yes, she's generally quite docile but, of course, she's extremely nervous and the slightest thing can upset her. You can always tell when she's in a bad mood – her nostrils flare and her ears go right back. Ah!—' He turned. 'Here's George laden with apples and – yes – an axe and a hammer.' He laughed, 'I must say, it looks a bit crude – not exactly delicate surgery – still, it may do the trick.'

He took the short-handled axe in one hand and the

hammer in the other and went down on one knee close to the bars.

'Here, Miranda,' said George enticingly. 'See what I've got for you.'

She gazed at him warily then the enormous neck came over the top and, as she took the apple and began to munch, Maurice said quietly, 'She's not near enough. See if you can make her move to the right.'

George shifted a little, held out another apple and she moved closer. Carefully placing the axe in position, Maurice waited a moment then, suddenly, down came the hammer in one sharp blow. Miranda's ears went back and she hesitated in the act of accepting the apple then, grabbing it quickly, she moved away, well out of Maurice's reach.

'Never mind,' said George. 'You've got quite a bit off. We'll have another go in a couple of days' time. It's a pity we can't use the hoof cutters but you'd never be able to manipulate them through the bars. This way, she doesn't really know what's happening.'

Maurice got to his feet and George went round to the back of the giraffe house to release the others.

A few minutes later a huge male, followed by a female and their year-old offspring, came swaying out and began wandering about while Maurice studied the young one closely.

'Yes, I'm afraid you're right,' he said at last. 'It seems to be hereditary. See—' he turned to me – 'Look at the mother.' The overpowering mama standing by her child began to move away and I saw that her left hind leg was turned out at the fetlock in a twisted fashion.

'Her knees are enlarged too,' said George, 'she was like that when she first came here but it hasn't deteriorated and it doesn't appear to bother her. Unfortunately, the youngster is going to be worse.'

'He's already getting a bit lame,' said Maurice and stood deep in thought for a few minutes. Then he said, 'You know, George, I think I'll try a course of calcium injections on him. I'll order the stuff I need and, if you can fix up a crush, we'll begin treatment next week. It will probably be a bit difficult to get him just where we want him so we'll have to allow a good bit of time. We don't want him to panic.'

'We'll work out something,' said George cheerfully. 'And now, I'd like you to have a look at an anaconda. It's got something wrong with its mouth.'

I shivered involuntarily. Snakes are my pet aversion.

'How big is it?' I asked anxiously.

'Oh, it's just a young one. About twelve feet long. Only half grown.'

He led us to the Reptile House and, at first, I thought I would wait outside. After a few minutes, however, my curiosity overcame my feelings of revulsion and I went in and saw George, his left arm outstretched, holding the rear end of the anaconda while his right hand was gripped firmly round the back of its head, holding it out for Maurice's examination. For a moment I couldn't understand how his arm could extend for twelve feet: then I realised that another man was holding the last few yards of the sinuous body. In the dim light it was hard to see the large black spots on the scaly greenish-brown skin but the cold, expressionless eyes sent a shiver down my spine.

'See,' said George, 'he's got this kind of fungus on his mouth.'

Maurice bent down and studied it closely.

'Mouth rot,' he said, 'I'll give you a liquid antibiotic which you can put on with a paint brush.'

Not waiting to see the creature put back into its living quarters, I went quickly outside and when the two men joined me, George said, 'Now for something completely different. We're going to do a spot of beaver hunting. I think the male has got something stuck in his throat – he can't close his mouth.' He turned to Maurice, 'You'll want your rubber boots – we'll have to wade in the pool to catch him.'

Maurice went back to his car and, when he returned with the boots, George handed him a net. Then he looked at the pool where a female beaver was swimming around with her two young ones.

'I think Poppa has gone into his den,' he said, 'I'll go round the back and push him out.'

150

Maurice waded into the pool and stood waiting with the net.

'Here he comes,' he said, and I saw a rather indignant beaver emerge reluctantly from his den in the bank: a strange-looking creature, about thirty inches long with a heavy body covered in glossy greyish-brown hair and an extraordinary tail. It was wide, scaly and black and looked rather like an oar. His face resembled that of an outsize guinea pig and I thought at first he would be easy to deal with, until I saw how quickly he dodged as soon as he caught sight of the waving net. Climbing over the barrier, George stood guard over the entrance to the den and Maurice chased the beaver from one end of the pool to the other. At last he trapped him and said, handing over the net to George, 'Hold him tight while I see if I can look in his mouth.' Then he added as the beaver snapped at him through the mesh, 'I think I can see the trouble. It's his lower big tooth. It can't meet the large front upper one. It's jutting back. It's very long. That's why he can't close his mouth.'

The furious animal began struggling even more wildly, biting at the net and getting so entangled that it was difficult to see how George would manage to hold him still. But, as Maurice produced a pair of what looked like wire-cutters from his pocket, George gripped the wet bundle so tightly that Maurice was able to get a hold on its mouth and cut the tooth in one swift movement.

'There you are,' he said, 'and I've still got my fingers.'

Turning the net upside down, George released the captive and, in a flash, he disappeared into his den. As the two men climbed out of the pool, Maurice said,

'I'll have to cut that tooth again in a few months' time because it will continue to grow.' He laughed, 'My veterinary skill this morning is rather like that of an old-fashioned "sawbones". What's next on the list?'

'The emu,' said George, 'We thought at first it had just gone lame but it's getting weak and there's obviously something else wrong.'

As we walked towards the enclosure Maurice asked, 'By

the way, have you managed to catch the thief who was stealing the ostrich eggs?'

George shook his head and grinned.

'No, we haven't managed to surprise him in the act but we don't think he'll come back again.' He turned to me, 'Did you hear about that little bit of trouble?'

I nodded. Maurice had told me that when the ostrich was laying one egg a day preparatory to incubating a clutch, the keeper found they were disappearing.

George chuckled, 'Well, she laid a third one and, this time, I took the egg away and replaced it with a coconut that I had shaved and painted white. It was gone the next morning and, since then, she has laid two more which have been left untouched.'

Maurice laughed, 'I'd love to have seen the thief's face when he examined his loot.'

'But why on earth should anyone want to steal a thing like that?' I asked.

George shrugged his shoulders.

'Some crazy collector or someone who thinks he can sell it. Or it might have just been a boy wanting it as a curiosity. Now—' he pointed, 'what do you think is wrong with Emma?'

The bird resting on the ground looked something like an ostrich except that she was covered right up to her small head with fluffy greyish-brown feathers and, as she got up, I saw that she was only about five feet tall. She took a few steps but she was swaying from side to side and she stumbled several times then sank down again and sat, looking straight ahead, as though resigned to her fate.

'She's running a temperature, obviously,' said Maurice. 'I'd better check it.'

George called to a keeper nearby and, taking out his thermometer, Maurice went into the enclosure with them. I didn't think Emma would offer any resistance but, to my surprise, as George and the other man rushed forward and grabbed her, she began to struggle wildly until, held by the neck and forced against the chain-link fence, she suddenly gave up the fight enabling Maurice to insert the thermometer.

'It's very high,' he said, then pulling his stethoscope from his pocket, he listened carefully to the bird's chest.

'I think it's a touch of pneumonia,' he said at last. 'I'll give her an antibiotic injection. Let's see – she's fairly heavy – about five cc.' He nodded to me and, opening his case, I filled a syringe and handed it to him. He put the needle quickly into Emma's thigh but she showed no sign of noticing it and immediately George and the keeper released their hold, she sank down onto the ground once more.

'She'll need at least three more injections,' said Maurice, 'and she'll take a bit more holding as she grows stronger. Let me know how she goes on.'

'Now,' said George, 'as I told you on the phone, the brindled gnu was found dead this morning. It was that young male that had been moved to fresh quarters some time ago. It seemed perfectly fit but, there it was, suddenly dead as a door nail. We've put it in our private yard for you to do a post-mortem to see if you can find out the cause of death. It was eating and behaving quite normally – no sign of illness whatever.'

'I'll just get my overalls,' said Maurice. When he came back from the car he was wearing his parturition gown which covered him from head to foot. George opened the door into the yard and I saw the gnu lying on the ground – a kind of antelope with pointed horns curved inwards, a black mane and a long black-tipped tail.

'I think I'll leave you to it,' I said, 'I'm not very keen on post-mortems,' and went off to the Zoo café for a much needed coffee.

As I sat drinking I looked out of the window at all the visitors milling around and reflected on the pleasure that a zoo can give to families with young children. Not that all the people here today had children with them. There were many groups of adults who, ignoring the amusements and entertainments provided for the youngsters, were content to wander from enclosure to enclosure just watching and commenting on the various species, obviously enjoying

153

themselves in a quiet way. It seemed a good means of passing a few hours leisure in order to relax and escape from the competitive world outside the Zoo gates.

Refreshed and rested I went back to join Maurice and George and met them just as they were coming out of the yard.

'It was pericarditis – fluid round the heart,' said Maurice. 'The poor creature must have been ill for some time but showed no symptoms. It's the old story – some animals disguise the fact that they're not well for fear of being set upon by the others. In the wild, they would go away and hide, but in captivity they can't do this so they adapt as best they can by pretending to be OK.'

He was washing his hands when, suddenly, from the direction of the elephant house, we heard trumpeting and squealing and Maurice looked up in amazement.

'What on earth—?'

George chuckled. 'It's all right. That's just Marjorie telling the world that her keeper has come back from his holidays. The whole time he was away she was miserable and sulky but he came back this morning and she's beside herself with joy. She's a very temperamental lady as you know and difficult to deal with but she has this terrific rapport with him and he can do anything with her.' He paused deep in thought for a few moments, then he went on, 'You know, it's a strange thing, this relationship between animals and their keepers. When we get a new man here it can be a bit difficult at first. Especially with an inexperienced one. They're usually young and, although they know they want to work with animals, they don't always appreciate the rather humdrum and often dirty work that has to be done. It's only a fairly small percentage that make the grade. They have to be dedicated. For the right kind of person it's a satisfying and worthwhile job. Sometimes they get fond of the most unprepossessing animals. One keeper was very attached to a particular baboon and always gave him a hot peppermint at night when he went off duty. When he went on holiday he left instructions to his replacement to do the same. But the baboon wouldn't take it from anyone else – threw it away –

and sat and moped. As soon as his keeper returned he was overjoyed, perked up and looked eagerly for his peppermint nightcap. Little things like that make animals happy.'

'It's sometimes a problem for me,' said Maurice, 'sorting out the physical from the psychological. Do you remember that time when Barbara the old elephant had us worried? Her appetite was erratic, her droppings weren't all they should have been yet her temperature was normal. I naturally thought she had been given something indigestible by one of the visitors but she didn't respond to my treatment. Then you discovered that there was trouble at night when she was being shackled by a new keeper.'

'I don't remember that,' I said. 'When did it happen?'

'Oh, it was a long time ago.' George frowned at the memory, 'I'll never forget catching that chap hitting Barbara with a broom. I asked him what the hell he thought he was doing and he said she was deliberately standing on her chain and refusing to budge. It turned out that she always did this when he had to shackle her. She didn't like him because he was rough and shouted at her so she just made things difficult for him. The other keepers never had any trouble. If she hadn't been so good-natured she could have really sorted him out and hurt him badly.' He looked at his watch. 'Well, that's all for now. No more problems, though I expect as soon as you've gone, some emergency will occur and I'll wish I'd kept you here a bit longer.'

Maurice smiled. 'I'd better get away while the going's good, then. Wait a bit – isn't that keeper trying to attract your attention?'

A man was running towards us and, as soon as he drew near, he called out, 'Mr Bowring   one of the monkeys has broken its arm.'

'Good lord!' George stared. 'How on earth—?'

'It's the Spot-nosed monkey,' said the keeper. 'No one saw it actually happen but he was probably cornered in a fight and must have got caught up in something. He's sitting on his own now and whimpering a bit. His arm is hanging loose and it looks broken to me.'

We hurried towards the monkey house and there was the

155

poor creature, nursing his arm and looking very sorry for himself. He was an attractive little fellow, distinguished by his peculiar nose which had a heart-shaped blob of white fur on the very end.

'I think I've got some plaster of paris in the car. Will you get him out?' asked Maurice, 'and I'll see what I can do.'

The keeper nodded and, picking up a net on a long pole, went into the enclosure. In a minute the monkey was enveloped and, although he protested at first, his wild chatterings had died down by the time we reached the annexe to the quarantine block.

Placing him on the table still in the net, the keeper held him there while Maurice prepared a syringe. Then, putting the needle into a muscle in the monkey's thigh, he waited for him to become unconscious. Then he took off the net and examined the arm.

'Yes, it's broken all right,' he said. 'Here – on the lower end of the humerus, just above the elbow. I'll have to put it in plaster. Will you give me a bowl of water, please?'

'I'll go and get the tin,' I said, and hurried off to the car. When I returned, Maurice took the roll of bandage and placed it in the bowl. Then, pulling the broken limb out straight, he lined up the bones and set the arm.

George said, 'Can I help?'

Maurice nodded. 'Yes. You hold it now and keep up the tension while I put on the plaster. I must be quick or it will go hard.'

Starting at the shoulder, he wound it right down the arm and the hand, covering the fingers, and then wound it back up to the shoulder again. A little more manipulation of the bones before the plaster hardened, an injection of antibiotic and, at last, he stood back satisfied.

'How long will he have to keep it on?' asked George.

'Three weeks, and of course he'll have to stay here for that time. When I take the plaster off – that's when your problems will begin.'

George nodded ruefully, 'Yes. We shall have to find somewhere else for him to live. Probably with a different species. Ah! well, another life saved. He would have died in the wild, I suppose.'

'It probably wouldn't have happened in the wild,' said Maurice, 'but you're quite right, of course – an injured animal has a poor chance of survival. The plaster is hard now so I'll put him in this cage and leave him to your tender care. I'll be in tomorrow to inject the emu so I'll have another look at him then.'

George walked with us to the car and then, just as Maurice was about to start up, he exclaimed,

'I nearly forgot — we need some more SA 37. About twenty pounds. Our stock is getting a bit low.'

Maurice stared in mock amazement. 'You certainly get through the stuff. Do you use it for your breakfast cereal with Yak's milk or something?'

George grinned amiably, 'How did you guess? That's why we're all so tough around here.'

'What on earth is SA 37?' I asked curiously.

'It's a powder containing minerals and vitamins which we add to the animals' food,' said George, 'It supplements their basic diet.'

'It must cost a fortune to feed them all,' I said.

George nodded. 'It's astronomical. We've had to cut some luxuries out since prices have risen so much. But they still eat better than they would if they had to hunt for food in the wild.'

'All this talk of food is making me hungry,' said Maurice, pulling the self-starter. 'See you tomorrow, George.'

'A very interesting morning,' I said when we arrived home. Maurice laughed.

'All rather elementary veterinary work,' he said, 'but the novelty lies in the variety of patients.'

'Very unappreciative patients. You certainly don't get much gratitude.'

'Oh, I don't know. Some of the more intelligent creatures seem to realise you're trying to help them. Anyway, it's very rewarding. And talking of rewards–' he went to the dresser and took out a bottle. As he handed me my glass, he said,

'Here's to the Zoo and all its inhabitants.'

I smiled.

'And here's to the Zoo's vet.'

Arthur Farrell was a retired gamekeeper we had known for many years. He lived in a tiny cottage on the edge of a wood with his one companion, an old Springer Spaniel, and whenever Maurice was passing he would call in to see him and listen with enjoyment to tales of the past.

But this morning Arthur had telephoned and, when I heard the sadness in his voice, my heart sank.

'It's Roy,' he said. 'I hoped he'd see me out but he's fourteen – that's ninety-eight, isn't it? – and he's very, very tired. Poor old boy, he tries to keep going but he can hardly get to his feet now, and it breaks my heart to see him struggling to follow me whenever I go outside. I'm afraid your good man will have to—' his voice broke.

'Maurice will come this afternoon, Arthur,' I said. 'I'm very sorry to hear that Roy is so weak. Perhaps—' but I couldn't hold out false hopes and the old man, his voice firmer now, said,

'Will you come with him and have a cup of tea with us? Roy likes it when I have company.'

The door of the cottage stood wide open when we arrived and Arthur, his dog at his feet, was sitting gazing towards the woods. As we approached they turned their heads slowly and the sadness in both pairs of eyes was enough to bring tears to mine.

'I'm very glad to see you, ma'am.' Arthur got up and put a kettle on the ancient old stove and the dog's eyes followed his master's every movement. 'You're pleased, too, aren't you, Roy?'

At the sound of his beloved master's voice, Roy's tail

159

thumped slowly up and down and then, as Maurice bent to stroke him, he tried to get up.

'It's all right, old boy,' said Maurice gently, 'you just lie down and rest,' and looked at him compassionately as he sighed and relaxed.

Arthur stood for a moment in silence then he turned to Maurice. 'Now, don't you go thinking that I'm hoping you can make him better. I know well enough that his time has come and I don't want to hold him back just for my sake. It would be much worse for him if I died first. Anyway, I don't suppose it'll be long before I follow him – that's if they'll let me in wherever he's going. But, first of all, I'd like to give you some tea.'

Taking a tin from the shelf he opened it and handed me a chocolate covered biscuit. 'I get these specially for Roy. He always has just one at tea time, but lately he's stopped eating. Perhaps he'll take one from you.'

I hesitated. 'I'd love to give it to him but I think you should this time.'

He nodded. 'You're right ma'am. It will be his last and it should come from me.'

Going down slowly on his knee, he held it out.

'Here's your biscuit, old boy. Eat it up, then you can have another one if you like.'

A lump rose in my throat as I saw the dog wag his tail feebly, take the biscuit in his mouth then, sadly, drop it on the floor beside him. As if to apologise to his master, he licked Arthur's hand lovingly and the old man stayed beside him for a full minute, stroking his head and whispering to him.

Then, getting stiffly to his feet, Arthur went over to the stove, made the tea and handed it round. We sat for a while in silence and then he began to talk.

'Roy and me have been together for fourteen years and he's given me the greatest happiness in the world, haven't you, Roy?'

The dog looked up and his dim eyes covered with the blue film of old age still seemed to radiate love as, once more, his tail went slowly up and down.

160

'He was a fine little pup when I got him and we were pals from the start. Weren't we, Roy?'

The tail went up and down again and, as the story of his life unfolded, master and dog seemed to be re-living it all over again.

As Arthur drew towards the end, I saw Maurice look quickly down at Roy.

'You've been the best dog in the world, haven't you, Roy?' Arthur's voice faltered and then I realised that, this time, the tail was still.

Bending down, Maurice felt the dog's heart, then he looked up.

'He's gone. The happiest death he could have had.'

Down on his knees again, the old man stroked his beloved dog and whispered something to him. Then, his face calm and peaceful, he rose to his feet.

'I hoped he'd go like that. Now, ma'am–' he looked at me and saw my tears, 'you just have another cup of tea and you'll soon feel better.'

Maurice said gently, 'Would you like me to take him away?'

'Oh, no. I've got a little place put aside for him.'

'Then let me help you. He's very heavy.'

The old man hesitated. I could see that he didn't want anyone else to touch his dearest friend but, realising he wouldn't have the strength alone, he said at last,

'We'll do it together.'

When they returned Arthur sank into his chair and looked down at the floor where Roy had so recently lain, listening to his master's loving voice.

Lifting his head he gave a long sigh, then, seeing my look of concern, he said, 'It's all right, ma'am. Don't you worry about me. I'm just glad my old dog had a happy death. I hope mine will be as easy.'

On our way home Maurice turned into the village.

'I think I'll call in and have a word with the district nurse. She's a client of mine and I'll tell her about Arthur. She'll keep an eye on him, I know.'

That evening, as we sat in the garden, Maurice said, 'I

almost envied Arthur giving his dog his last happy memories. I would have loved to have been able to do that to old Bill.'

I remembered then, how when Maurice had joined the Army at the outbreak of war, and before we had even met, he had owned a Springer Spaniel that was as close to him as Roy had been to Arthur Farrell. He had once told me that his worst moment after he volunteered had been the realisation that he would have to leave Bill. His mother had looked after him devotedly but the poor dog pined badly. He spent most of his time upstairs in Maurice's room, lying under the bed with an old cap his master had worn when they had spent happy hours together in the country.

His sad whimperings were almost more than Maurice's mother could bear and, one day, she took the cap away. But Bill became so desperately unhappy, searching everywhere, that she gave it back to him. Consoled a little, Bill gradually settled down. Then Maurice came home on leave and the dog went simply mad with joy, and they spent every moment together until the day came when Maurice had to return to his regiment. He put the cap in Bill's basket and told him he would soon be back. But it was the final parting because Maurice was sent overseas and, before he returned, Bill had grown so old that he had to be put to sleep.

'Even now,' said Maurice, looking into the distance, 'I feel a pang of regret that I couldn't have been with him at the last.'

I thought of all the dogs who had loved us so faithfully, Merlin and Major, Jason and Robin and then looked down at Robert who, sensing his master's sadness, put a gentle paw on his knee.

'Man's best friend,' I said.

'I agree,' said Maurice, 'though there's an awful lot of anti-dog propaganda going around nowadays. It's the latest neurosis. People are getting worked up to a ridiculous degree. I met a man the other day who wanted to keep a dog, but his wife was dead against it because she was convinced that pets would pass on dreadful diseases. I told her that this thing has been magnified out of all proportion and that the few – very, very few – dangers that do exist can be entirely avoided by responsible ownership. Ordinary cleanliness, regular immunisation and regular worming.' He paused and grinned ruefully. 'She said I had an axe to grind and, of course, I have but not just because I'm a vet. I feel very strongly that animals help to keep us all sane.'

We had just finished morning surgery the following day when the telephone rang and Maurice answered it. He listened for a minute, then he said,

'I'm glad. It was what he wanted. Thank you for telling me.'

He put down the receiver and looked at me.

'That was the district nurse. Arthur had a stroke last night. He never recovered consciousness and died this morning.'

I put two cups of coffee on the table and we sat drinking for a few moments in silence. Then I said,

'One can't be sad about it. It was a merciful thing to happen. Perhaps he's with his old friend now – you never know.'

Maurice smiled. 'It's a nice thought,' he replied. 'But, of course, it wouldn't be the same.'

'What do you mean?'

'Well – ' he looked amused, 'I shouldn't think there's much work for a gamekeeper up there, would you?'

Chapter Twenty-four

Maurice frowned as he read through the list of calls he had to do after morning surgery.

'These are going to take nearly all day,' he said, 'just when I was hoping to get down to some paper work.'

'You mean the accounts?'

'Those too. But I've got some Health Certificates that must go out today and some Ministry of Agriculture forms to fill in.' He paused for a moment then glanced at me. 'Do you think—?'

I nodded. 'Of course. I'll do what I can.'

He looked relieved. 'That's fine. The most urgent things first – the accounts can wait.'

'They always do,' I said, 'but I'll make a start on them if I can. The only trouble is your writing – talk about deciphering a secret code!' I picked up a sheet of paper from his desk. 'This one for instance – a Health Certificate for fifty – for heaven's sake – it looks like fifty "goldfish"!'

'That's right. Fifty goldfish going to Nigeria.'

I stared. 'What an extraordinary thing. How on earth do they travel?'

'They'll fly, of course. Swimming would be rather tricky because of the difficulty of getting them all to go in the right direction.'

I laughed. 'Ask a silly question and I get that kind of answer. I meant, how do they transport them?'

'They travel in large plastic bags – no, I'm not being funny, the bags are about the size of pillow cases – in about eight inches of water. Then oxygen is pumped in until they look like great big balloons. Then the bags are put in cardboard cartons. Any more questions? I'm late already.'

I waved him away and, still smiling to myself at the idea of fifty little goldfish with labels round their necks, all swimming madly in the general direction of Africa, I settled down to the typewriter, hoping fervently that I would not be interrupted.

For half an hour I worked steadily. Then the telephone rang.

'Mrs Brook here,' said a voice I knew well. Glancing at the clock, I bet myself that it would be at least five minutes before this particular lady would get down to the reason for her call. 'I'd like your advice. I don't know whether to get Mr Bowring to come here or whether to come to the surgery. The trouble is that my husband and I are going out this evening and I have so many little jobs to do. You know how it is, although I expect, with a husband like yours who is always popping in and out, you can rely on him for help in emergencies. What I always say is, if there is a man in the house, you might as well make use of him. Little things take up so much time, don't they?'

I was about to break in but she was in full spate now, so resigning myself to the inevitable, I waited patiently.

'As soon as Bobby comes in, I get him to empty the waste bins, water the pot plants and see if I've run out of anything in the grocery cupboard. Men just don't realise what there is to do in a house. Why, only the other Thursday – or was it Monday? No, it couldn't have been because—'

She paused for a second and I seized my opportunity.

'Do you want my husband to call to see your dog, Mrs Brook?'

'Oh, no. Hamish is fine. He takes up a great deal of my time, though. I often say to Bobby, you don't realise, I say, what a lot of work that dog makes. In and out of the garden all day and, each time, I have to wipe his paws in case he brings any mud into the house—'

'Mrs Brook – ' I was getting desperate, 'I'm very sorry, but I shall have to hurry you up. There's someone at the door. Could you tell me quickly if you want my husband to call?'

'What? Oh, yes. Well, it's my cat – look, you just go and answer the door then I can tell you about it afterwards.'

'I'm afraid I can't do that. It would take too long. I have to give a grocery order. Now, if you would like my husband to call it will have to be late in the afternoon, he's extremely busy.'

'But I'm not sure if I want him here. It's Tabitha's ear, you see. She's shaking her head a lot and, last time, Mr Bowring gave me some powder to puff in. But I've finished it now so I thought I could call at the surgery and collect some more.'

'That's fine,' I said, 'so we'll see you either this evening or tomorrow morning.'

'Oh, dear. I'm afraid I can't come then. It may have to be tomorrow evening.'

'Tomorrow is Mr Bowring's half day. No evening surgery.'

'Then what shall I do? Perhaps he'd better call after all. But not this afternoon – I shall be too busy. You see, I have to get ready for going out this evening. You know how it is – a special dress and my hair to do and—'

'Tomorrow morning, then,' I said firmly. 'I'll tell him.'

'I suppose that will be the best time, though, after having been out late—'

'Good.' I cut her short. 'Now I really must go.'

As I wrote down the message I reflected wryly that Mrs Brook was well named. She certainly went on for ever and was probably still babbling away quite unaware that I had hung up.

My concentration rather impaired, I began work again, but ten minutes later, I really did hear someone at the door. This, I decided, was a judgment on me for having invented an imaginary tradesman and, reluctantly, I went to investigate.

To my surprise, I saw a large, dishevelled woman in her mid-thirties, surrounded by what seemed a whole tribe of small children all leading or clutching animals of various kinds. At a glance I saw three puppies, two hamsters and a very small kitten, and shaking my head, I said,

'I'm sorry, but surgery is over for this morning and Mr Bowring is out on his calls.'

'Oh, that's all right.' A broad smile allayed my fears that all these animals needed instant veterinary attention. 'We were just passing so I thought I'd drop in to ask a question. It's about some guinea pigs I bought for the children. I got one for each child and the man assured me they were all males. But now I'm not so sure. Two of them are very fat and getting bigger every day. If I bring them to the surgery tomorrow morning, do you think Mr Bowring will be able to tell me if they are females and going to have babies?'

'Oh, yes,' I said, 'I'm sure he'll be able to sort that out for you.' I smiled at the children. 'What a lot of pets they have. Do they always take them along when they go out with you?'

She gave a warm, easy chuckle as she gathered her brood together. 'It keeps them happy. They've got more animals at home. Rabbits, white mice – the trouble is I can never say no, so they're turning the house into a zoo. Tell Mr Bowring I called, will you? Lily Clutton is the name.'

Before I could sit down again the telephone rang once more and a brusque voice asked, 'Does Mr Bowring attend horses?'

'Yes,' I replied. 'He does a lot of horse work.'

'Ah, but does he *know* anything about them?'

I stared at the receiver, unable to believe my ears. At last I said, 'Well, that's for you to decide, isn't it?' and felt my temper rise as the voice went on,

'I've heard good reports of him but you can't believe everything you hear. I don't know whether to get him to examine my mare or not. We're new to the district and where we lived before we had a very good vet. Well, he wasn't much good at first but I got him trained eventually and he always did what I wanted.'

'I can't guarantee that my husband will do everything you want,' I said rather sharply, 'but I can assure you that he will do what is best for the animal.'

'Hmm.' There was a long pause. 'Well, of course, if you're the vet's wife, you're bound to be prejudiced, aren't you? Anyway, I have a dog who needs a booster injection so he can come over and do that. Then I can give him the once over and decide whether to have him for the mare. I'll give you the address.'

I took it down then smiled grimly to myself. 'I'm sorry, but I'm afraid you live too far outside my husband's practice. It would involve too much travelling. I think you would be better advised to find a vet nearer to you.'

'I don't see that distance comes into it. I'm perfectly willing to pay. Anyway, I'll ring again and see what your husband has to say. After all, it's for him to decide, isn't it?'

Muttering indignantly to myself, I went to make a strong cup of coffee. Then, with a firm resolve not to get involved in any more long conversations, I settled down again. Luckily, I was left in peace and, by the time Maurice came in for a quick lunch, I had done all the urgent work and was well into the accounts.

'I've had a hell of a morning,' he said, 'but I've managed to get most of the calls done. Only a couple left over for this afternoon – that is, if nothing else has come in.'

'Only Mrs Brook tomorrow morning, though she may change her mind again. And a lady is bringing in two guinea pigs tomorrow morning. She has lots of children, lots of animals, and lots of problems, it seems, caused by the fact that she can never say no.'

Maurice grinned. 'Ah, that's Lily Clutton. How many children has she got now?'

'Well, I saw five,' I said, 'but now I come to think of it, I believe there's another on the way.'

Maurice laughed. 'Well, she'll have to start saying no soon. Is that all?'

'Only a perfectly objectionable woman whom I've done my best to discourage.'

I told him the story over lunch and he said, 'You coped with her very well. I'm certainly not going to be anyone's tame vet.'

Once more the telephone rang and Maurice got up to answer. He was such a long time that, at last, I went and stood by him, listening curiously. Finally he said, 'I'll come this afternoon,' and although I could hear the caller still talking, he put down the receiver. Then he turned and grinned at me. 'Mrs Brook. She's decided she wants me this afternoon after all. The gas man is going to be there tomorrow and she can't cope with more than one person at a time. God! How that woman does dither.'

A thought struck me. The gas man.

'That reminds me,' I said, 'I've got to fix up a day to have the boiler serviced. I'd better do it now before I forget.'

It was when I was trying to arrange a date that I realised I had mislaid my diary. 'Hold on a minute,' I said, and searched frantically in my handbag. 'Ah, here it is,' I said. 'No, I'm sorry, you can't come on Friday after all – I've a dental appointment. Monday, perhaps – no, that's no use. Could you come on Wednesday? Not possible? Well – Thursday? Oh, but that's my husband's half-day so I'd rather not. Could you make it Tuesday? Of course I'm not undecided – I'm simply trying to find a free day. Yes, the boiler does need servicing and I do want you to do it – that's why I'm ringing up. Tuesday then? The only thing is – oh, all right. Tuesday afternoon. Couldn't you make it in the morning? Yes, I know you're a busy man but so am I – I mean a busy woman. Oh, very funny but I'm not joking. So you'll come on Tuesday morning – sorry, afternoon. Of course I won't forget and go out shopping. I shall have to do that in the morning, won't I? That's why I would have preferred you to come in the morning so that I could have gone shopping in the afternoon. Yes, I've got it straight. Tuesday afternoon. Goodbye.'

I turned away from the telephone and saw Maurice standing behind me with a most peculiar expression on his face.

'What's the matter?' I asked.

'Oh, nothing, nothing,' he said hastily. 'I was just thinking about Mrs Brook.'

'Mrs Brook? Why – you can't mean that I—?' I stopped and then, as he began to laugh, I said indignantly, 'Ridiculous! I'm not like her at all. I know my own mind. I don't dither.' I paused and thought back for a moment. 'Well, not very much.'

170

'It's all right,' said Maurice comfortingly, 'you aren't quite as bad as Mrs Brook. Not yet, anyway.'

Chapter Twenty-five

Maurice's birthday is in August and, after carefully studying the calendar, I was pleased to see that, this year, it would fall on a Sunday.

'Oh, good,' I said, 'You'll be able to please yourself during the day and we will all enjoy your birthday dinner in peace. Now – what would you like to have for the main dish?'

'Oh, I don't know – something simple. Wait a moment, though – how about having that peahen in the freezer?'

'Good heavens!' I stared at him incredulously, 'do you really think you would like it?'

'Yes, rather.' For once, Maurice appeared interested in food. 'That is – not if you don't want to bother with anything so fancy. Perhaps you'd like it better if I took you all out to dinner.'

'It's your birthday,' I said, 'and if you would like the peahen then we'll have it. Mind you, I haven't the faintest idea how to cook it but I'll look it up in "Mrs Beeton".'

A few days later I went to the freezer and hauled out the – to me – rather repellent bird that had been given to us about a month ago. As I placed it on a dish to thaw out, I remembered how it had come into our possession.

Maurice had returned from a farm one morning carrying a very large dead bird which he laid on the kitchen table.

'What on earth is that?' I asked, 'something from the Zoo?'

He grinned, 'It's a peahen. A present from Mr Needham over at Thetford farm. I am assured that these birds are very good to eat.'

'I didn't know the Needhams bred peacocks for the table. Surely there can't be much demand for them nowadays?'

'They don't breed them. This one appeared out of the blue. Apparently, the other morning their little daughter came running into her parents' bedroom saying there was a vulture sitting on the wall outside her window. When her father went to look he saw the back of a big bird that he recognised as this peahen. The family went out to investigate and it came down from the wall and followed them round into the farmyard where they gave it some corn. At first, they were very amused and supposed it would eventually go away but, after a time, some of their free range hens came into the yard looking for their usual tit-bits and went into a panic at the sight of a monster devouring their food. So the Needhams went to the telephone and rang up the Zoo and several other places where they thought peacocks might be kept. But no one had lost a bird and no one wanted it either. They were a bit nonplussed at this so they went out again intending to shoo it away and, this time, they found trouble. A mother hen, with her brood of about eight baby chicks only a few days old, was practically in hysterics because the peahen had already pecked two babies to death.'

'Oh, dear,' I said. 'Well, I can guess the rest.'

Maurice nodded. 'Yes. Mr Needham was a bit apologetic about it but he said he had no option but to shoot the wretched bird. Anyhow, there he was. Landed with a dead peahen and his wife firmly refusing to have anything to do with it. She said she could never bring herself to cook, let alone eat such a murderous creature. It seemed a pity to waste it so he offered it to me.'

Looking down at the limp body on the table I was inclined to agree with Mrs Needham but Maurice said, 'I'll pluck it and put it in the freezer. I believe it was considered a great delicacy in the old days.'

I nodded rather doubtfully, thinking of one or two other things that were considered delicious in our grandparents' time. Marrow-bones dished up with special forks for digging out the succulent content, roast larks and boiled sheep's brains. I decided I had no great yearning for the old days and took no further interest in the peahen which, at the bottom of my capacious freezer, soon became well covered and forgotten.

But a birthday request could not be ignored, so, with half an hour to spare, I went in search of 'Mrs Beeton'.

The copy I possess has been handed down through my family. It was given to my great-grandmother when she got married and studied fervently by all her descendants. Although it was now ragged and worn it was still one of my greatest treasures providing mostly amusement nowadays but still containing gems of culinary interest.

I searched in the index for peahen and there it was, complete with illustration. A very big bird lying on a dish with its long neck and head curled round itself and even the eyes left in. I shuddered. Nothing so gruesome would appear on my table. Then I remembered thankfully that Maurice had already cut off the head.

I began to read the recipe: 'A peahen', Mrs Beeton stated, 'makes a magnificent dish. The fowl must be young' – Oh dear! Maurice had guessed its age at about two years. Well, I'd just have to cook it very slowly – 'The head', continued the great authority, 'must be enveloped in paper with the feathers on while the bird is cooking, then garnish with watercress and arrange the neck and head tastefully, as in our illustration.'

I shook my head. Even John and Margaret, with their liking for exotic foods, would pale at such a grisly sight. I decided to cook it as I would a turkey, with all the trimmings. Then, if it should be tough, we could fill up with the 'etceteras'.

I began turning the pages, marvelling at the enormous amount of food our ancestors consumed. A horrid picture of a pig's face on a plate, with the caption: 'A nice breakfast dish', caused me to move hastily on to the section for soups and my attention was caught again.

'A useful soup for benevolent purposes as made by the editress in the winter of 1858 for distribution among a dozen poor families in the village.' It contained at least eighteen ingredients including half a pint of beer. I hoped the villagers enjoyed it and, resolving to try it out on the family on some future occasion, I studied a scale of servants suited to various incomes. According to that, I should be employing a cook, an upper and under housemaid, a kitchen maid, a scullery maid and a manservant. I sighed. Those were the days! Then common sense took over and I remembered my grand-mother's tales of a houseful of servants but also a nursery full of children, many of whom did not survive.

I closed the book. Life was better nowadays for everyone.

The birthday dinner was a great success. We had it in the garden and, although the peahen was a little hard, it went down very well, helped by a bottle of champagne – the last of half a dozen bottles given to us by a client in the wine business.

But suddenly, as we sat drinking coffee, revelling in the warm summer evening and watching the swallows swooping low over the fields, the telephone rang.

'I'll go,' I said, going indoors fully prepared to fend off anyone who wanted Maurice unnecessarily.

'Oh hello, George,' I said. 'Don't tell me you want Maurice at the Zoo at this hour?'

'No, don't worry. I meant to ring him earlier but I forgot. It's just to ask him if he will drop in some Aureomycin tomorrow when he's passing.'

I was very relieved. 'I'm so glad he hasn't got to go out this evening. You see, it's his birthday. You'll never guess what we had for dinner – a peahen!'

'That's interesting,' George began to chuckle, 'I believe one of ours went missing about a month ago.'

'What? Oh dear!' Quickly I told him how it had come into our possession, adding 'the Needhams rang the Zoo at the time and were told it didn't come from there.'

'I expect they spoke to someone who wasn't up to date.' George evidently found it highly amusing. 'Don't let it bother you – we've got far too many peacocks and hens as it is.'

He rang off still laughing and I put down the receiver and went back to the family.

I gave Maurice the message but said nothing about the peahen. George would enjoy pulling his leg tomorrow but

176

today was his birthday. It was, I felt, hardly the moment to tell the doctor that he had just eaten one of his patients.

Chapter Twenty-six

Maurice was late again for breakfast. John and Margaret had already left to catch their bus and I was beginning to worry about morning surgery when, at last, I heard his car.

When he came in I looked at him askance. Although he always has a clean-up at a farm after any dirty work, it was plain to see that, on this particular occasion, his rough-and-ready toilet had been extremely hasty. His hands were clean and that was about all. There were streaks of blood on his face that had escaped the quick rinse with cold water, straw clung to his jacket and trousers and wisps of hay peeped out from behind his ears. His general appearance was that of a tramp who had spent the night in a barn and ended up in a fight with the farmer.

'You wouldn't believe the trouble I had with that calving,' he said. 'The cow had twins, the second one was dead and I had a hell of a job to get it out.' He paused and looked down at the breakfast table. 'No time for that, I'm afraid. A bath is more important.'

'Both,' I said firmly, and when, about twenty minutes later, he sat down under protest to toast and honey, I poured out two cups of hot coffee. When he had finished, I said, 'George rang from the Zoo. He knows you are going to start on the calcium injections for the giraffe this morning but he asked if you could get there earlier than originally planned. The American Bison has gone down and they can't get him up and there are several other animals with problems.'

'It's going to be a long session then. Let's hope nothing urgent comes in.'

'Would you rather I stayed home to deal with the telephone?'

'Oh, no. I'll get it transferred to the Zoo. You'd like to come, wouldn't you?'

'No need to ask,' I said. 'It sounds as though it will be an interesting morning.'

'It always is,' said Maurice.

Luckily for us it was a quiet surgery and, with no operations to do, we set off for the Zoo in good time.

'The American Bison,' I said, 'that's a buffalo, isn't it? Would you say it was dangerous?'

Maurice laughed,

'I think that would be a fair description. They're very large, very powerful beasts but, as this particular one is down and unable to get up, I expect I'll be able to treat it.'

When we arrived at the bison's enclosure, accompanied as usual, by George, the sick animal was lying on his side and, seeing us, he tried to rise, grunted in pain and went down again, rolling and kicking.

Maurice looked at him for a few moments. 'His stomach is distended and blown up with gas. A bad case of colic. I'll give him an injection. When did he last eat?'

'He hasn't touched anything for two days,' said George, 'but he only went down this morning.'

He was indeed, as Maurice had said, a powerful-looking animal. His face and the front half of his body were covered in dark brown shaggy hair and his thick neck rose to a hump. His head, with its short curved horns, and his shoulders seemed out of proportion to his hind quarters; and his huge, ugly face was made even fiercer-looking by a dark beard under his chin.

'That's his mate next door,' said George. 'We've separated them for the moment. She's the original bearded lady.' I looked and laughed. Sure enough, although she was much smaller and not so fierce in appearance, she had a very handsome beard indeed.

Maurice opened his case, took out a syringe and a bottle and, while he prepared the injection, George armed himself with a pitchfork.

180

'I'll give him a jab with this if he turns on you,' he said.

Maurice grinned. 'Well, be careful. I don't fancy those prongs in me. You look much more dangerous than he does at the moment.'

They went into the enclosure and Maurice began talking quietly and making soothing noises but the bison grunted angrily and, rolling his eyes, tried to get up, luckily without success. George stood behind, very much on the alert, and suddenly Maurice banged the needle into the animal's rump, fitted on the syringe and, in about ten seconds, completed the injection. Just in time, as it happened, for once more the bison began to roll and kick.

'That will take about half-an-hour,' said Maurice when they came out. 'I'll come back and look at him when we've done the giraffe.'

This time we went round the back of the giraffes' enclosure and I stood in a passage where, through the chain-link, I could see into the sleeping quarters. The young giraffe was alone, walking around restlessly, probably wondering why he wasn't out in the sunshine with the others. He looked slightly apprehensive as Maurice, with George and the keeper, went in and began to urge him gently towards the crush.

This was a kind of swinging gate in iron framework, with a wheel at one end and a hinge on the other, folded back against the wall. At first, the giraffe moved forward obediently until he was past the hinged end but then, suddenly suspicious, he retreated. The men backed and waited quietly then, almost imperceptibly, began to ease him once more in the right direction. At last, unawares, he walked into the trap, the door was swung round and bolted and he was jammed up against the wall. He tried to struggle and kick but he was too constricted and, realising he was helpless, he resigned himself to his fate and stood quite still. The door was cleverly designed with lots of small holes at various heights so that different parts of the animal's body could be examined and, if necessary, injected. Maurice carefully chose a convenient one but, owing to lack of space, the needle would not go into the giraffe. He experimented for a few moments, holding the needle in various ways, then, at last, with a very big push he managed to penetrate the tough hide.

'That's it,' he said. 'You can let him go now.'

George undid the bolt, eased the door open, and the giraffe, looking extremely affronted, swayed off to the farthest corner of his lofty house.

'I'll give him one a week,' said Maurice, as we went out into the open, 'possibly for about six weeks. Watch him carefully for signs of improvement.'

The keeper nodded and then asked, 'Will you have a look at the adult male now? He's been having difficulty with eating. He's dribbling a lot and there seems to be something wrong with his tongue because, when he's offered something, he goes to take it but doesn't put his tongue out properly.' He took a banana out of his pocket. 'Look – this is one of his favourite treats.'

The enormous male, standing against the chain-link, put his head eagerly over the top. Hesitantly, the long tongue came partly out of his mouth and took hold of the banana, but almost immediately dropped it onto the ground beside him. Another try and, as his head bent down, Maurice said, 'I don't think it is his tongue. His neck is puffy. Compare it with one of the others. His glands are swollen and it hurts him to put out his tongue. He needs an injection of antibiotic.' He paused. 'It will be impossible to drive him in now so I'll come along tomorrow morning. Keep him in for me, and in the meantime here's some stuff to put in his drinking water.' He looked at his watch. 'I'd like to go and have a look at that bison now.'

A keeper was standing watching him and he turned as we approached.

'He seems much better,' he said, 'he got to his feet five minutes ago. He's salivating a lot, though.'

'That's the effect of the drug,' said Maurice. 'It shows it's working. What we want now is—ah, that's it – look.'

The bison, standing with his back to us, began to strain slightly and then, without any difficulty, passed a large lump of dung.

182

George looked pleased. 'That's fine. He's on the mend. Do you think he'll need another injection?'

'I sincerely hope not. He should gradually recover completely. But keep an eye on him. It's a pity we can't give him a drench as one would to a domestic bull but, with no ring in his nose to control him, it's not possible.'

As we turned away George said, 'A nasty thing happened just before you arrived. A man and his wife came up to me and said they had seen a boy throwing stones at the flamingos. When they went to stop him he ran off and they were unable to catch him. Then they went back to the birds and saw that one of them had been injured. Hopping on one leg with the other hanging limp.'

We went over to the lake where the beautiful exotic-looking birds lived and their gorgeous salmon-pink plumage gave a great splash of colour to their surroundings. The poor injured flamingo stood alone at the water's edge, hunched up with his feathers fluffed out, motionless and miserable.

Maurice said angrily, 'Yes, that leg is definitely broken. I'd like to get my hands on the young devil who did it.'

George nodded in agreement. 'Is there anything you can do?' he asked.

'I'm afraid not.' Maurice shook his head regretfully. 'You know how we've tried in the past and it never works. The blood supply is very scanty and, even if you can get the bones to join, the tendons that operate the toes never run smoothly over the callous and the bird is permanently lame. Just the same as in a horse.'

George pursed his lips. 'Only one thing for it then?'

'Yes. It's kinder to put it down now. I'll give it an overdose of anaesthetic.'

He prepared a syringe and George went in to catch the bird. It began to hop away in alarm but, almost immediately, collapsed on to the ground and George picked it up gently, tucked it under his arm and carried it outside.

Suddenly, in spite of the sadness of the moment, I was reminded irresistibly of the illustration in *Alice in Wonderland*, when, playing croquet with the Queen of Hearts, Alice

183

has great difficulty in managing the flamingo which she has to use as a mallet.

Maurice saw my involuntary smile and stared at me in surprise. 'Alice in Wonderland,' I said briefly.

'I don't see what—' He looked completely bewildered then, as he glanced at George coming towards us, light dawned.

'You have a macabre sense of humour,' he said, but I saw his mouth twitch.

He was serious however when he followed George into a shed and I waited outside while he put the poor bird out of its misery.

A short time later they both reappeared and I asked, 'Where are we off to now?'

'To the Malayan Sun bears,' said George, 'there are three of them together – all females – and the third one has only recently arrived. They seemed to get on very well until yesterday evening. Then they had a bit of an argument when they went into the passage leading to their sleeping quarters. It's a bit narrow there and the first two ganged up on the newcomer. It was probably only a momentary tiff but the new one was bitten rather badly.'

As we set out for the other side of the Zoo we passed the monkey section and George said, 'By the way, we've arranged new accommodation for the little Spot-nosed monkey. When you took the plaster off the other day we put him over there with two females. He seems to have settled down well. You'd never know he'd had a broken arm. He's full of beans.'

He pointed,

'See – there he is. Oh ho, he's seen you coming. Look – he's nipped behind those nettles.'

Sure enough, while the other two monkeys continued to climb around, Maurice's ex-patient had discreetly taken cover. But he was not completely invisible, for every now and then, from behind the clump of greenery, the little face with its startling white nose jerked up and then bobbed down again as soon as he saw us.

'He won't forget you quickly,' laughed George. 'That's

gratitude for you. See – there he is again – popping up and down like a jack-in-a-box.'

We remained watching for several minutes, then one of the others came forward and sat on the ground in front of us. I was fascinated as she moved her head from side to side in quick jerky movements with her intelligent eyes fixed on us searchingly.

'They really are most attractive little creatures,' I said. 'I could watch them for hours.'

'No time for that,' said Maurice, 'I've got a tricky job ahead if that Sun bear needs stitching.'

George led us round to the back of the bears' enclosure until we came to a padlocked door. As he took out a key and opened up I said, 'This is new territory to me. I've never been here before.'

He grinned, 'You're privileged. No member of the public is ever allowed round here. It's too dangerous.'

Suddenly I saw what he meant. The sleeping quarters were covered by a door which he now pulled up and there, only a few inches away, was the bear.

'Don't go any nearer,' he warned. 'Those claws could come out in a flash.'

He turned as a keeper joined us who said, 'More trouble. I've put the American Black bear next door for Mr Bowring to examine.'

He opened the compartment beside the first bear.

'He's suddenly begun salivating like mad. Looks as though he's got something stuck in his throat.'

The bear was standing close to the bars, shaking his head from side to side with saliva pouring from his mouth and covering his shoulders and half his body. In spite of the mess he was in I could see he was very big with a coat of dense black shiny fur. His neck was so short that his head, with its rounded ears, seemed to come straight from his shoulders and, at the end of his short legs, thick paws carried terrifying long claws.

'Can he swallow?' asked Maurice.

'Yes,' said the keeper, 'but he brings everything up immediately afterwards.'

185

'Let's try him with something now.'

The man took an apple from his pocket.

'He's been eating these,' he said, throwing it between the bars.

The bear lurched over, picked it up, chewed and swallowed. Then, a minute later, he vomited.

Maurice looked puzzled.

'Well, it's obviously not his throat – more likely the gullet.' He stood for a few moments deep in thought then said, 'You say he's been eating apples. I wonder—' He paused and looked around. 'You know, there are lots of wasps about now. I believe he's swallowed one and got stung either in the stomach or oesophagus.'

George nodded. 'That might well be. The fruit gets left around and he may have picked up an apple with a wasp inside.'

'I'd better deal with him first,' said Maurice, 'I'll have to dart him with a dose of anti-histamine. That means I'll have to use a barbless needle so that we can knock it out. Unfortunately they're not very reliable because they sometimes fall out too soon and you can never be sure that the whole dose has been administered.'

At that moment the bear, still streaming saliva, turned his back on us and Maurice said softly,

'Good. That's just how I want him.'

Swiftly he loaded up the dart gun and we all stayed motionless as he went quickly up to the bars, took aim and fired.

To my surprise the bear took no notice whatsoever but I could see the dart was sticking in his haunch.

'Now,' said Maurice, 'we must get it out.'

The keeper took a long pole, passed it through the bars and tried to knock the dart out of the thick fur. It took several minutes because, not wanting to attract the bear's attention, he had to poise the pole right over the dart, and just as he was about to strike downwards the bear chose that moment to shake his head violently. But eventually he knocked it down on to the floor and then, very carefully, worked it back until Maurice was able to put his hand in and grab it out.

'Damn!' he said. 'The dose is still there. We'll have to try again.'

He recharged the gun and fired again and the dart landed almost in the same place. The same procedure was followed and this time the dart was empty.

'Well, the dose is in,' said Maurice, 'and that's all I can do for now. The salivating should stop in a few hours if my diagnosis is correct. If not, ring me up and I'll try something else.'

Suddenly the bear turned, ambled back to the bars and stood gazing at us. He was so close that I thought aloud, 'He looks quite harmless, doesn't he? I can imagine that if a child stood here, it would be an awful temptation to put in a hand and stroke his nose.'

'He'd have him in a split second,' said George. 'Bears never alter their expression – never give any warning. It's impossible to judge their mood. Members of the cat tribe and other carnivores will demonstrate their feelings by snarls and growls but these fellows are inscrutable. They are also completely fearless.' He turned to the next compartment. 'Now the Sun bear is not so dangerous. She's much smaller – the smallest of all the bears in fact – but of course like the rest of them, quite unreliable.'

She was right at the back of her den now, lying down. 'She's looking very sorry for herself,' Maurice remarked. 'I'll have to dart her with anaesthetic. Then you can pull her out here in the open and I can examine her.' He paused. 'What do you suppose she weighs?'

'It's difficult to be accurate,' said George. 'About a hundred pounds? She's only about half the size of the Black bear.'

Maurice shook his head.

'Not as much as that, I'm sure. I don't want to kill her with an overdose. I should think about eighty-five pounds – let's compromise at ninety.'

I tensed a little as I always do when Maurice loads the dart gun with the anaesthetic that is instantly lethal to man and leant forward to make sure that he had the antidote ready in case he should spill a drop on his own skin. At last it was ready and, once more, he fired.

'Bang on!' he said. George laughed. 'You're a crack shot. It's a good job you are – those darts are expensive.'

We stood waiting for the bear to lose consciousness and after about ten minutes Maurice said,

'Right! She's under now. Let's have her out.'

The door was opened, she was dragged out and, as she lay on the ground at our feet, I looked at her with interest. This bear's black coat was short, with a white 'V' on the chest. Her face was broad with a fawn muzzle and her small eyes gave her a slightly Asiatic appearance.

'Why are her front legs so bandy?' I asked curiously.

'She's a tree climber,' said George, 'but her legs are short and she uses those front ones like arms to curl round thick branches.'

Maurice finished his examination and stood back.

'Two nasty bites on her back,' he said, 'large round holes about the size of an old penny, and her left hind foot is badly chewed up.'

Opening his case, he threaded a suturing needle with heavy gut and then began to sort out the bits of muscle that were sticking through the wounds. After a while, he shook his head. 'It's hopeless trying to join up all these torn ends. They're too mangled. I'd better let nature do it in her own time.'

He took the needle and began suturing the skin but, as he pushed, it bent double.

He frowned, 'Talk about tough old boots,' he said and selected another needle but the result was the same. Another needle and, this time, he managed to penetrate the skin but had to take a pair of forceps to pull it through. It was a slow difficult job but, at last, he was satisfied.

'Those sutures will dissolve in about twenty days,' he said to George, 'by which time the wounds should have healed. But the foot is impossible to suture. I'll have to let it drain, give an injection of antibiotic and let you have some in powder form to put in her drinking water. It will eventually heal that way. Now—' he turned to the keeper, 'she must be

188

shifted to a spare den and kept there until she's completely fit again. I'll give her the antidote now and she'll be round in about ten minutes.'

From around the corner the keeper produced a barrow, the bear was lifted in and Maurice gave the injection. The man was off like a flash and George chuckled.

'No need to run,' he called out. 'Mr Bowring said ten minutes – not ten seconds.'

The keeper half turned, 'Better to be safe than sorry,' he said and rushed away, not willing to take any chances.

'Only one more case,' said George, as he padlocked the gate behind us, 'it's the camel with diarrhoea. He's no better.'

'Hmm.' Maurice looked rueful. 'That's the two-humped job that nipped me in the shoulder last time I examined him.'

'That's the boy,' George chuckled, 'it's funny how he seems to dislike you. He gets on fine with his keeper.'

'His keeper doesn't stick needles into him,' retorted Maurice. 'I quite understand his resentment but I don't much care for his way of expressing it. Now, let me see—' He paused. 'Ah, yes. I sent off the sample of faeces to the laboratory and I got the report back yesterday. A very high worm content. In fact, it's shot right up since the last check a month ago. So it's no use treating him by mouth. I'll have to give him a very large dose – about twenty cc.'

The Bactrian camel's usually disdainful expression seemed to become even more scornful when he caught sight of Maurice, and George said, 'I'll just go and rustle up some extra help. His keeper is having a day off, so what with that and your presence, he'll probably be a bit difficult. We'll have to rush him.'

He returned with four men, one of them carrying a wire mesh frame about the size of a door, and opened the gate. Then they charged in and before the startled camel had time to realise what was happening, he found himself pressed up against the wall. Bellowing and roaring, he tried at first to break away but in the end, recognising that he was helpless, he contented himself with glaring at Maurice who stood waiting with a syringe. There was an ominous pause and a keeper, guessing what was coming, put up his hand to turn

189

the camel's face away. Unfortunately for him, he only partially succeeded and the camel, playing his trump card, ejected the contents of his stomach and sprayed the unlucky keeper with a shower of evil smelling semi-digested food.

The man swore, George chuckled and Maurice moved in to give the injection. 'I can hardly see which is camel and which is keeper,' he said. 'let me know if I miss because if I stick it into one of you, I'll have to fill the syringe again.'

But there was no yell from any of the keepers and, as soon as the injection had been given, they all made for the gate. Suddenly the camel was free but he remained where he was for a few moments, still spitting and roaring, until, realising at last that the battle was over, he stalked away.

As George recovered his breath, Maurice said, 'He'll have to be kept in his paddock on the concrete. Don't let him go on the grass until this trouble has cleared up.' He looked at his watch. 'I'll just nip down to the Sun bear and make sure she's properly round from the anaesthetic and I'll meet you in the bar. I think we deserve a drink.'

As George and I strolled along I said, 'I must just have a look at the Orang-Utans. They fascinate me. Whenever I see them, they've always got their arms round each other and they're always smiling.'

'Well,' George smiled too, 'that's the way their mouths are shaped. But they certainly are very fond of each other. They're also the most intelligent of all the apes.'

We stood for a while by the railings in front of the water barrier dividing the apes from the public and, as usual, the male and female orangs sat smiling together. Ugly yet attractive creatures, covered by long auburn hair, they squatted at the edge of the water, contemplating the world outside with good-humoured interest.

The wide moat sloping down to a depth of about eight feet, ran along the front of three separate sections, with the orangs in the first division, the chimpanzees in the middle and the gorillas at the end. Although I could see the other apes playing around, every now and then emitting their peculiar cries, the orangs remained quiet, in a peaceful world of their own.

'We gave all the apes a little intelligence test the other week,' said George. 'We took twelve white plastic bins about a couple of feet tall, with flat tops and bases. We gave three each to the chimps, the gorillas and the orangs. They were all out here in the open. The gorillas, being the most destructive, tore their bins to pieces in no time at all and that was that. The chimps of course, showed off like mad – carried the bins around, sat on them, put them on their heads and pranced about getting lots of laughs from the public, which pleased them immensely. But the orangs just sat and looked at their three bins and we decided they weren't even interested. They did nothing for three days then, on the fourth, Tuan, the male, suddenly got up, took one bin, went along to the shallow part of the moat and placed it carefully in the water. Then he went back for the second one and, to our utter amazement, he stepped carefully on to the first, placed the second one a short distance ahead and returned to get the third. Using the first two as stepping stones, he put the third one still farther ahead in the water and as near as possible to the side of the iron railings where they curve round. He was just about to jump onto it and reach out for the rails when he overbalanced and fell into the water. Of course he panicked, then immediately forgot his clever plan and scrambled back to dry land. But if he had succeeded, he would have been up the railings and outside in a flash. Their minds work slowly – very slowly – but they do work things out. Unfortunately for Tuan, he couldn't overcome his fear of water. They all hate it, you know.'

Maurice joined us as we went into the bar. 'The Sun bear has come round nicely,' he said, 'so that's OK. Now – what will you have?'

For about twenty minutes we talked, or rather, I listened as Maurice and George exchanged anecdotes about the inmates of the Zoo, and then we set off for home.

'I feel as though I've done a whole day's work in one morning,' said Maurice. 'Thank goodness no urgent calls have come through.'

I remembered then that he had been to a difficult calving case before breakfast.

'You must be tired,' I said, 'why don't you try to have a rest this afternoon? I'll do my dragon act on the telephone and put off unnecessary calls till tomorrow.'

'A very good idea,' said Maurice. 'I'll sit in the garden and watch the bees slaving themselves to death for me.'

When he was installed in the hammock after lunch, I looked out, saw him reading the newspaper, saw the newspaper fall onto the grass, and shut the window near the telephone so that he would not hear it if it rang.

It did, of course, but only once. The caller was a lady who said she just wanted some information.

'I know your husband does dogs and cats,' she said, 'and, I suppose, farm animals. But does he see to hamsters, guinea pigs and rabbits?'

'Oh, yes' I said. 'He has lots of clients who keep pets like that.'

'And budgies?'

'Those too. Animals, birds, reptiles – you name it – he treats them all. Anything, in fact,' I added with wifely pride, remembering the inhabitants of the Zoo, 'anything from tortoises to tigers.'